Dessert Recipes

117 Desserts That Are Tasty, Quick & SO Easy to Make!

by Olivia Rogers

Copyright © 2017 By Olivia Rogers
All rights reserved. No part of this book may be reproduced in any form without permission in writing from the author. No part of this publication may be reproduced or transmitted in any form or by any means, mechanic, electronic, photocopying, recording, by any storage or retrieval system, or transmitted by email without the permission in writing from the author and publisher.
For information regarding permissions write to author at
Olivia@TheMenuAtHome.com
Reviewers may quote brief passages in review.

Please note that credit for the images used in this book go to the respective owners. You can view this at: TheMenuAtHome.com/image-list

Olivia Rogers
TheMenuAtHome.com

Table of Contents

1. Banana Pudding *8*
2. Coconut Cream Pie Bars *8*
3. Cool Lemon Bars *9*
4. No-Bake Cheesecake *10*
5. Coconut-Berry Fro-Yo Pops *11*
6. Strawberry Mango Crumble *14*
7. Strawberry Margarita Pops *15*
8. Banana Bread Ice Cream Sandwich *15*
9. Mint Chocolate Chip Ice Cream *16*
10. Peanut Butter Pie Pops *17*
11. Chocolate Ice Cream *18*
12. Chocolate Peanut Butter Banana Icebox Cake *19*
13. Lemon-Blackberry Yogurt Pops *20*
14. Raspberry Trifle *21*
15. Ginger Fruit Salad *22*
16. Yogurt with Walnuts & Plum Compote *22*
17. Cookie Icebox Cake *23*
18. Grilled Peaches with Yogurt *24*
19. Key Lime Pops *25*
20. Macedonian Fruit Salad *25*
21. Macaroon Ice Cream Cake *26*
22. Chocolate Muffin Sandwiches *27*
23. Ginger Peach Ice Cream Pie *27*
24. Raspberry-Orange Sherbet Cake *28*
25. Lemon Ices *29*

26. Mango Sorbet _____ 30
27. Ice Cream Snow _____ 30
28. Lime Coconut Sorbet_____ 31
29. Creamy Avocado Pops _____ 32
30. Chocolate Almond Bars _____ 32
31. Fresh-Fruit Popsicles_____ 33
32. Peanut Butter Cookie Dough Bars _____ 34
33. Cookies and Cream Melt-Aways_____ 35
34. Orange Cream Freezer Dessert_____ 36
35. Ice Cream Sandwich Cake _____ 37
36. Pink Lemonade Pie _____ 37
37. Layered Melon Kiwi Jell-O Cups _____ 38
38. Banana Split Fluff Salad_____ 39
39. Raspberry Sorbet _____ 40
40. Banana Chocolate Ice Cream_____ 41
41. Cherry Vanilla Coca-Cola Ice Cream Float_____ 41
42. Chocolate Cake Ice Cream Truffles_____ 42
43. Frozen Grasshopper Squares _____ 43
44. Ice Cream Sundae Cookie Cups _____ 43
45. Pineapple Coconut Frozen Yogurt _____ 45
46. Hazelnut Mocha Ice Cream_____ 45
47. Layered Berry Vanilla Soft Serve_____ 46
48. Snickerdoodle Ice Cream Sandwiches _____ 47
49. Lime Creamsicles_____ 49
50. Greek Yogurt Fudgesicles _____ 50
51. Chocolate-Dipped Pear Popsicles _____ 50
52. Salted Caramel Milkshake _____ 51

53. Coconut Granita 52
54. Chocolate Frosting Shots 53
55. Strawberry Crème Truffles 53
56. Frozen Cookie Dough Bites 54
57. S'mores Ice Cream Sandwiches 55
58. Sweet Potato Ice Cream 57
59. Raspberry Coconut Chia Ice Pops 58
60. Caramel Candied Almonds 59
61. Double Chocolate Chip Cookies 59
62. Frozen Chocolate Chip Cookie Dough Yogurt 60
63. Nutella & Cream Popsicles 61
64. Banana Bread Brownies 62
65. Candied Blood Oranges 63
66. Blackberry Cabernet Popsicles 64
67. Tangerine Prosecco Sorbet 65
68. Candied Pumpkin and Yogurt Kataifi 65
69. Honey Lemon Custard with Fruit 66
70. Poached Pears with Pepper Ice Cream 67
71. Hot Cocoa with Peppermint Ice Cream 69
72. Buttermilk Panna Cotta with Apricot and Candied Fennel _ 70
73. Frozen Ginger Vanilla Yogurt with Peach Compote .. 71
74. Cinnamon Bundt Cake 72
75. Peach Rosé Gelée 73
76. Spiced Squash Pie with Pumpkin Seed Crumble 74
77. Purple Rice Pudding with Rose Water Dates 76
78. Ginger Cream 77
79. Italian Ice Cream Sandwiches 78

80. Mint Watermelon Ice Cubes	78
81. Chocolate Oatmeal Pie	79
82. Curry Ginger Sugar Cookies	81
83. Cherry Almond Chocolate Bark	82
84. Salted Caramel Risotto	83
85. Chocolate Dipped Candied Orange Peels	84
86. Strawberry Black Pepper Truffles	85
87. Strawberry S'mores	86
88. Honey Molasses Glazed Oranges	87
89. Walnut Amaranth Cookies	87
90. Rose Prosecco Pops	88
91. Greek Yogurt Topped with Cherries & Almond Syrup	89
92. Berry Plum Pudding	90
93. Cranberry Pistachio Oatmeal Ice Box Cookies	91
94. Grilled Peaches in Herb & Lime Syrup	92
Special BONUS Recipes!	93
95. Peanut Butter Eggs	94
96. Fruit Pizza Pie	95
97. Coconut Muffin Cake	96
98. Mini Carrot Cake	97
99. Lemon Bars	98
100. Snickerdoodle Bars	99
101. Sugar Cookies	100
102. Breakfast Carrot Waffles	100
103. Coffee Cream Cheese Cake	101
104. Chocolate Tart	103
105. No Bake Key Lime Pie Bars	104

106. No Bake Gingerbread Cookies & Creamy Frosting _____ 105
107. Pumpkin Pie Cheesecakes _____ 106
108. Apple Crumble Cupcakes _____ 107
109. Traditional Strawberry Short Cake _____ 107
110. Fudge Brownies & Cream Cheese Frosting _____ 108
111. Chilled Peanut Butter Pie _____ 109
112. Vanilla Angel Food Cake _____ 110
113. Chocolate Truffles _____ 111
114. Chilled Creamy Orange Tarts _____ 112
115. Coconut Cream Pie Bars _____ 113
116. Berry Pudding _____ 114
117. Fruit Cobbler _____ 115
Final Words _____ 116
Disclaimer _____ 118

1. Banana Pudding

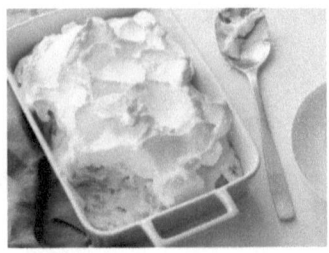

This chilled banana pudding is perfect for a hot summer day.

Ingredients

- About 48 Vanilla Wafers
- 6-8 bananas (sliced)
- 2 cups milk
- 1 (5 oz.) box instant French vanilla pudding
- 8 oz. cream cheese
- 14 oz. sweetened condensed milk
- 12 oz. frozen whipped topping (thawed)

Method

1. Arrange a layer of Vanilla Wafers in the bottom of a baking dish (13"x9"x2"). Arrange a layer of banana slices on top. In a bowl, blend together pudding mix and milk.

2. In a separate bowl, beat together cream cheese and condensed milk until a silky consistency is achieved. Whisk in whipped topping. Stir this mixture into the pudding mixture until blended. Pour pudding over bananas. Cover with another layer of Vanilla Waffers. Refrigerate 1-2 hours.

2. Coconut Cream Pie Bars

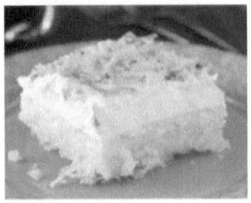

These scrumptious little treats have a refreshing coconut flavor.

Ingredients

- 8 oz. Vanilla Wafers (crushed)
- 24 Vanilla Wafers
- 6 tbsp. butter (melted)
- 8 oz. cream cheese
- ¼ cup sugar
- 3 cups whipped cream (divided)
- 1 (5 oz.) box vanilla pudding (prepared)
- 1 ½ cups coconut flakes (toasted, divided)

Method

1. In a bowl, combine crushed wafers and butter, and spread across the bottom of a baking dish (9"x13") in an even layer. Let set in the fridge.

2. In a separate bowl, beat together cream cheese and sugar until smooth. Gradually whisk in 1 cup of whipped cream. Spread over chilled crust. Arrange a row of wafers around the edge of the dish (with wafers standing upright). Return to fridge.

3. Whisk together pudding and 1 cup whipped cream. Carefully fold in ¾ cup coconut flakes until combined. Spread this evenly over the cream cheese layer. Spread remaining 1 cup of whipped cream evenly over pudding layer. Sprinkle remaining coconut flakes on top. Let chill 6 hours. Cut into bars to serve.

3. Cool Lemon Bars

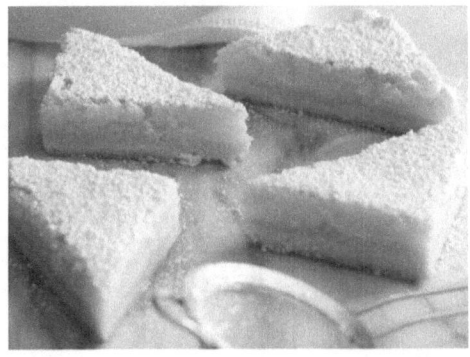

These citrusy sweets get a wonderfully crunchy texture from chopped hazelnuts in the crust.

Ingredients

- 1 cup butter (softened)
- 2 cups flour
- ¾ cup powdered sugar
- ½ tsp. vanilla extract
- ¼ cup chopped hazelnuts
- 1 tbsp. fresh grated ginger
- ¼ tsp salt
- 1 egg yolk
- 8 oz. cream cheese
- 8 oz. mascarpone cheese
- 28 oz. sweetened condensed milk
- 4 large eggs
- 1 tbsp. lemon zest
- 1 cup fresh lemon juice
- 6 tbsp. boiling water
- 1 tbsp. unflavored gelatin

Method

1. Preheat oven to 350°F. Line a baking dish (9"x13") with aluminum foil. Allow 2" of aluminum to hang over each short side. In a bowl, beat together butter, sugar, and vanilla until creamy. Gently beat in flour, ginger, salt and egg yolk. Stir in hazelnuts until combined. Spread across bottom of baking dish in an even layer. Bake 10-15 minutes. Let cool.

2. In a bowl, beat together cream cheese and mascarpone until creamy. Add condensed milk until blended. Add one egg at a time, beating each well. Add lemon juice and zest. Beat until thickened.

3. In a small bowl, whisk together gelatin and boiling water until dissolved. Let cool 5 minutes. Beat gelatin into lemon mixture. Pour mixture into dish. Refrigerate 8 hours. Cut into bars.

4. No-Bake Cheesecake

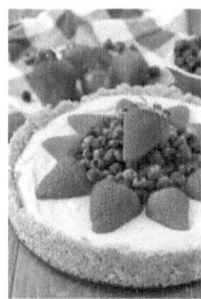

This effortless cheesecake is bursting with fresh blueberry flavor.

Ingredients

- 5 oz. Vanilla Wafers (crushed)
- 4 tbsp. butter (melted)
- 8 oz. cream cheese
- ¾ cup sugar
- 1 tsp vanilla extract
- Zest from 1 lemon
- 2 ½ cups blueberries
- Whipped cream and more blueberries to serve

Method

1. In a bowl, mix together crushed wafers and butter until combined. Divide mixture between 2 (4.5") pie dishes. Press into an even layer on bottom and along sides (about halfway up the sides). Freeze 30 minutes.

2. In a processor, pulse together cream cheese, lemon zest, sugar, and vanilla until smooth. Add blueberries. Pulse until blended. Divide filling evenly between each dish. Cover and chill overnight. Serve with a dollop of whip cream and blueberries on top.

5. Coconut-Berry Fro-Yo Pops

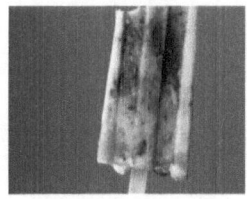

Frozen yogurt is already a great summer dessert, but these Popsicle versions make it an even more fun and convenient treat.

Ingredients

- 2 cups mixed berries
- ¼ cup sugar
- Juice from 1 lemon
- 1 cup plain Greek yogurt
- ½ cup powdered sugar
- 1 tbsp. coconut extract
- ½ cup unsweetened coconut flakes

Method

1. In a processor, pulse together berries, sugar, and lemon juice until smooth. In a bowl, whisk together yogurt, sugar, and coconut extract until smooth.

2. Pour alternating layers of berry mixture and yogurt mixture in popsicle molds. Insert sticks. Freeze for 8 hours. Remove from mold and dip into coconut flakes before serving.

Read This FIRST - 100% FREE BONUS

FOR A LIMITED TIME ONLY – Get Olivia's best-selling book *"The #1 Cookbook: Over 170+ of the Most Popular Recipes Across 7 Different Cuisines!"* absolutely FREE!

Readers have absolutely loved this book because of the wide variety of recipes. It is highly recommended you check these recipes out and see what you can add to your home menu!

Once again, as a big thank-you for downloading this book, I'd like to offer it to you *100% FREE for a LIMITED TIME ONLY!*

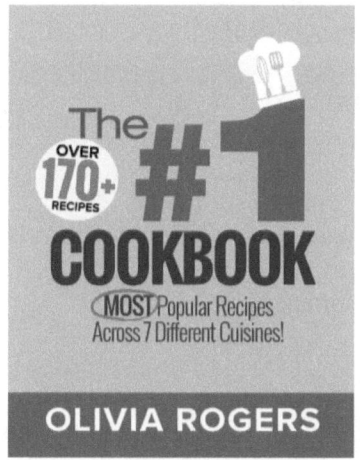

Get your free copy at:

TheMenuAtHome.com/Bonus

6. Strawberry Mango Crumble

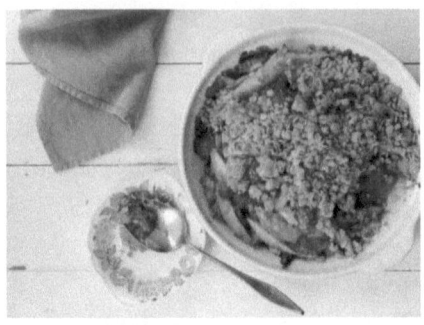

This simple dessert has all the flavors of summer.

Ingredients

- 3 mangos (peeled, sliced)
- 2 cups strawberries (quartered)
- 1 tbsp. sugar
- 2 tbsp. fresh lemon juice
- 1 ¼ tsp cinnamon (divided)
- ¼ tsp nutmeg
- 1 tsp grated ginger
- 3 tbsp. flour
- Salt
- 1 ½ cups flour
- 1 ½ cups rolled oats
- 1 cup brown sugar
- 10 tbsp. butter (softened)

Method

1. Preheat oven to 375°F. In a bowl, gently mix together strawberries, mangos, 1 teaspoon cinnamon, nutmeg, ginger, 3 tablespoons flour, lemon juice, and a dash of salt. Pour into a deep pie dish (9").

2. In a bowl, stir together oats, brown sugar, flour, a pinch of salt, and remaining cinnamon until mixed. Gently massage butter into mixture with a fork until clumpy. Spoon crumbly mixture over fruit filling. Bake 1 hour. Serve with ice cream.

7. Strawberry Margarita Pops

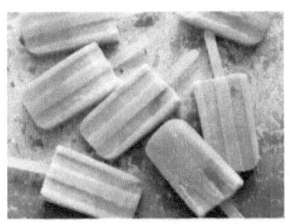

Liven up your backyard barbecue with these fun margarita pops.

Ingredients

- 1 cup fresh lime juice
- ½ cup water
- ½ cup triple sec
- ¼ cup tequila
- ½ cup sugar
- 1 pine strawberries (quartered)

Method

1. In a bowl, blend together water, triple sec, lime juice, tequila, and sugar until dissolved. Set aside 8 pieces of strawberry. Add rest to blender. Pulse until smooth. Stick a strawberry piece on the end of each Popsicle stick.

2. Pour margarita mix into popsicle molds. Insert sticks (strawberry side first). Freeze for 4 hours.

8. Banana Bread Ice Cream Sandwich

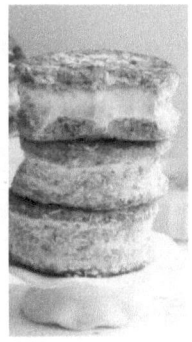

This recipe puts a twist on two classic desserts: banana bread and the ice cream sandwich.

Ingredients

- 3 ripe bananas
- 1 ½ cups flour
- 1 tsp baking soda
- ¾ tsp salt
- 2 eggs
- ½ cup sugar
- ½ cup butter (melted)
- 2 tbsp. olive oil
- ½ cup buttermilk
- 1 ½ tsp vanilla extract
- Ice cream (your choice)

Method

1. Preheat oven to 350°F. In a bowl, mash bananas until smooth. Whisk in buttermilk and vanilla extract. In a separate bowl, whisk eggs, sugar, butter, and oil until frothy. Stir banana mixture into egg mixture.

2. In another bowl, mix together flour, salt, and baking soda until blended. Gradually add flour mixture to banana mixture until combined. Pour into a greased loaf pan. Bake 1 hour. Let cool.

3. Prepare a grill of medium-high heat. Cut banana bread into 16 slices. Grill slices 2-3 minutes per side. Let cool. Spread about 1 cup of ice cream evenly on each sandwich to make 8 sandwiches. Chill sandwiches 1 hour.

9. Mint Chocolate Chip Ice Cream

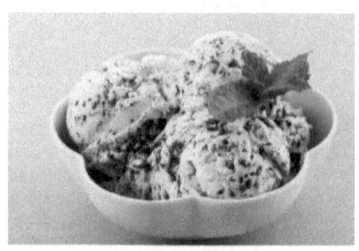

Make this classic summer treat from scratch in your own kitchen!

Ingredients

- 3 cups half & half
- 1 cup heavy cream
- 8 large egg yolks
- 9 oz. sugar
- 1 tsp. peppermint oil
- 3 oz. dark chocolate (chopped)
- Ice cream maker

Method

1. In a medium pan over medium heat, stir together cream and half & half and allow to simmer. Remove from heat.

2. In a bowl, whisk egg yolks together, and then slowly whisk in sugar. Stir in 1/3 of cream mixture in spoonfuls until well blended. Pour in the rest of the cream mixture in one batch. Return mixture to the pot and place on low heat. Stir often until mixture thickens.

3. Pour into a bowl and let rest for 30 minutes. Stir in peppermint oil. Chill in fridge for 4-8 hours. Pour mixture into an ice cream maker with dark chocolate. Prepare according to directions.

10. Peanut Butter Pie Pops

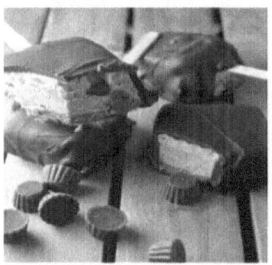

These peanut butter pie pops are both satisfying and refreshing.

Ingredients

- ½ cup graham cracker crumbs
- ¼ cup pretzels (crushed)

- ¼ cup sugar
- 1 tbsp. cocoa powder
- 3 tbsp. melted butter
- 12 oz. cream cheese
- 8 oz. peanut butter
- 4 oz. powdered sugar
- ½ tsp. salt
- 1 tsp. vanilla extract
- ¼ cup roasted peanuts (chopped)
- 1 ½ cups heavy cream
- ½ cup toffee pieces
- 6 oz. dark chocolate (chopped)

Method

1. In a bowl, combine graham cracker crumbs, crushed pretzels, cocoa powder, and sugar. Mix in butter until combined. Beat cream cheese until smooth. Beat in peanut butter, salt, vanilla extract, and powdered sugar until mixture is light and fluffy. Stir in peanuts until evenly distributed.

2. In another bowl, whip heavy cream into firm peaks. Fold cream into peanut butter mixture in ½ cup batches. In the popsicle mold, add alternating layers of peanut butter mixture, toffee pieces, chocolate, and graham cracker mixture until filled. Insert sticks. Freeze overnight.

11. Chocolate Ice Cream

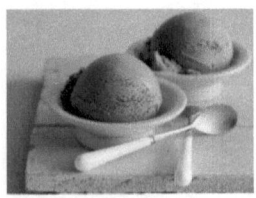

Make your own sinfully delicious chocolate ice cream with this recipe.

Ingredients

- ½ cup unsweetened cocoa powder
- 3 cups half & half
- 1 cup heavy cream

- 8 large egg yolks
- 9 oz. sugar
- 2 tsp. vanilla extract
- Ice cream maker

Method

1. In a medium pot over medium heat, whisk together 1 cup half & half with cocoa powder until combined. Add cream and remaining half & half. Stir until simmering. Remove from heat.

2. In a bowl, whisk together yolks and then slowly whisk in sugar. Whisk cream into the egg mixture in 1/3 cup batches. Pour back into pot. Place over low heat. Stir until mixture thickens. Pour into a bowl. Let rest for 30 minutes. Stir in vanilla extract. Cover and chill for 4-8 hours. Pour into an ice cream mixer and prepare according to directions.

12. Chocolate Peanut Butter Banana Icebox Cake

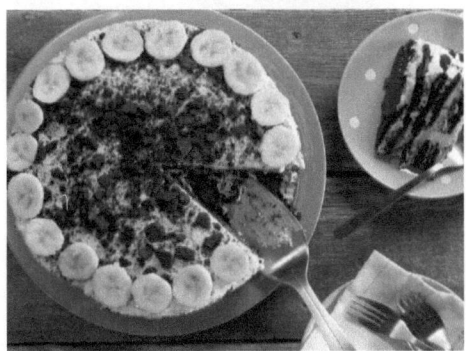

This no-bake cake combines the rich flavors of peanut butter, chocolate, and banana.

Ingredients

- ½ cup peanut butter
- 2 ½ cups heavy cream (chilled, divided)
- ½ cup powdered sugar
- 1 ½ tsp. vanilla extract
- 5 ripe bananas (sliced)
- 2 (9oz.) packages chocolate wafer cookies

Method

1. In a large bowl, whisk together peanut butter and ½ cup cream until fluffy. Set aside. In a separate bowl, whip remaining cream with sugar and vanilla extract into firm peaks. Fold about ½ cup whipped cream into peanut butter mixture. Add peanut butter mixture into whipped cream mixture in 3 batches until well combined to create filling. Set aside.

2. Arrange a layer of wafers in a 9" pie dish. Spread a layer of peanut butter filling on top. Add a layer of banana slices. Repeat layering until ingredients are used. Cover and chill for 4 hours.

13. Lemon-Blackberry Yogurt Pops

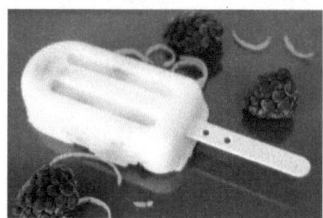

These cool popsicles are a perfect balance of tangy and sweet.

Ingredients

- 1 lemon
- ½ cup water
- ½ cup sugar
- 1 ½ cups plain Greek yogurt
- 2 cups blackberries (halved)

Method

1. Peel lemon. Set lemon and peel aside for another use. In a small pot over medium-high heat, stir together water and sugar until dissolved. Gently stir in lemon peels, and simmer 5 minutes. Let cool. Strain syrup into a bowl. Chill.

2. Stir yogurt into syrup until well combined. Stir in blackberries. Fill popsicle molds with yogurt mixture. Insert sticks. Freeze for 3-4 hours.

14. Raspberry Trifle

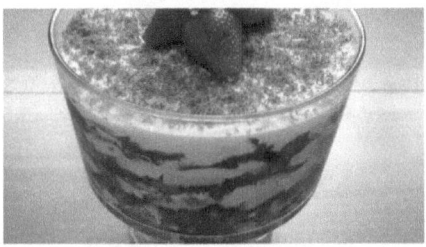

This simple custard dish is bursting with cool raspberry flavor.

Ingredients

- 9 egg yolks
- 4 cups whole milk
- ½ cup Sugar
- ½ vanilla bean (seeded)
- ¼ cup water
- 1 cup raspberry jam
- 1 cup heavy cream
- 1 cup dry sherry
- 2 loaves pound cake (sliced)
- 3 cups frozen raspberries (defrosted)
- 2 cups fresh raspberries

Method

1. In a bowl, whisk together milk, yolks, ¼ cup sugar, and vanilla seeds. Pour into a double boiler and set over medium heat, whisking constantly for 30 minutes without letting it boil to create your custard. Remove from heat and refrigerate 2 hours. Bring water to a boil in a small pot. Remove from heat. Stir in jam. Dip one side of each pound cake slice into the sherry. Arrange a layer of pound cake on the bottom of a large clear bowl.

2. Pour a thin layer of custard over the slices (just enough to cover). Spoon in a few teaspoons of jam mixture. Sprinkle in some defrosted raspberries. Repeat layering until ingredients are used. Poke a knife through the top in a few places. Top with fresh raspberries and whipped cream (if desired). Chill for 1 hour.

15. Ginger Fruit Salad

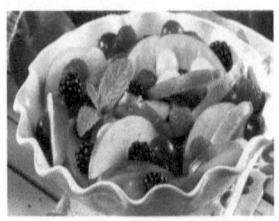

This jazzed up fruit salad is brimming with tropical flavor.

Ingredients

- ¼ cup sugar
- 1 (3") piece ginger (peeled, chopped)
- Zest from 1 lime
- 1-pint strawberries (quartered)
- 2 kiwis (peeled, quartered)
- 1 mango (cut into chunks)
- 1 pineapple (cut into chunks)
- 1 papaya (cut into chunks)
- 1 handful fresh mint (chopped)

Method

1. In a small pot, boil water, lime zest, ginger, and sugar until dissolved. Remove from heat. Refrigerate until chilled. Strain syrup into a large bowl. Add fruits. Toss to coat. Chill 1 hour. Garnish with fresh mint before serving.

16. Yogurt with Walnuts & Plum Compote

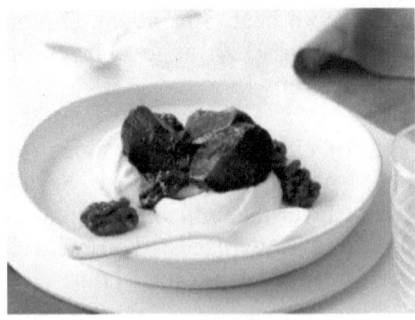

Yogurt gets a makeover with this irresistible plum and walnut topping.

Ingredients

- 5 ripe plums (pitted, quartered)
- 3 tbsp. maple syrup
- 2 tbsp. water
- Juice from ½ lemon
- 1 cinnamon stick
- 1 ¼ cups toasted walnuts
- 6 cups vanilla Greek yogurt

Method

1. In a pot over medium-low heat, cook plums, lemon juice, maple syrup, water, and cinnamon stick. Allow to simmer while you stir, and then reduce heat to low. Let cook 15 minutes. Remove from heat.

2. Stir in 1 cup walnuts. Divide yogurt into bowls. Spoon plum compote over the top. Sprinkle with remaining walnuts.

17. Cookie Icebox Cake

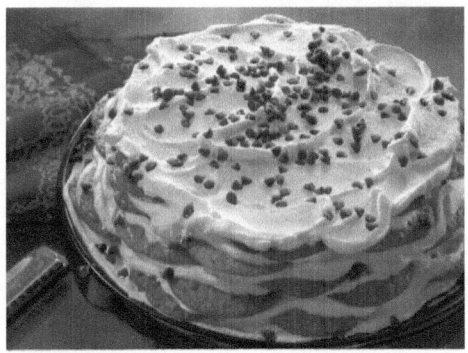

This simple no-bake cake is perfect to whip up for a potluck or barbecue.

Ingredients

- 40 chocolate wafer cookies
- ¾ cup sugar
- ¼ cup water
- 3 cups whip cream

Method

1. Pour sugar into a medium pot so that it forms a pile in the center. Slowly add water without letting sugar hit the sides of the pan. Cook over high heat. When sugar starts to color, gently stir. Let it become dark. It will smoke a bit.

2. Once darkened, reduce heat to medium-low and add 1 ½ cups cream. Gently whisk until caramel is dissolved. Stir in remaining cream. Strain into a bowl. Cover and chill. Whisk 2/3 of the chilled caramel cream to soft peaks.

3. Line a loaf pan (8"x4") with plastic wrap. Add a layer of cream to the bottom. Add a layer of cookies. Repeat layering until ingredients are used. Chill 3 hours. Invert cake onto a platter. Whip remaining cream into firm peaks. Spread over the cake.

18. Grilled Peaches with Yogurt

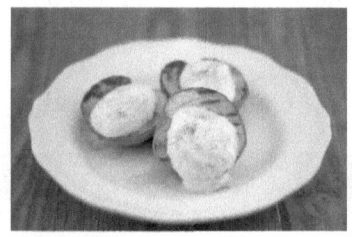

This dessert is healthy and elegantly simple to make.

Ingredients

- 12 peaches (halved, pitted)
- 2 tbsp. olive oil
- Salt
- 2 cups plain Greek yogurt
- ¼ cup honey
- 1 cup fresh mint (chopped)

Method

1. Prepare grill for high heat. Brush oil on peach flesh. Sprinkle lightly with salt. Place peaches (flesh-side down) on grill. Cook 1-2 minutes.

Transfer to plates and serve with a large dollop of yogurt. Drizzle with honey and sprinkle on fresh mint.

19. Key Lime Pops

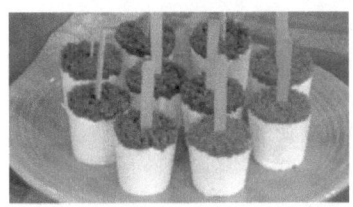

This recipe gives you a cool new way to enjoy the refreshing flavor of key lime pie.

Ingredients

- 1 (14oz.) can sweetened condensed milk
- 1 cup half & half
- ¾ cup fresh lime juice
- 2 tsp. lime zest
- Salt
- 3 cups graham crackers crumbs

Method

1. In a bowl, whisk together condensed milk, half and half, lime juice, zest, and salt until well combined. Divide mixture into Popsicle molds. Freeze for 1 ½ hours. Insert sticks. Freeze 4 hours. Spread graham cracker crumbs on a plate. Press popsicles into crumbs until coated on all sides.

20. Macedonian Fruit Salad

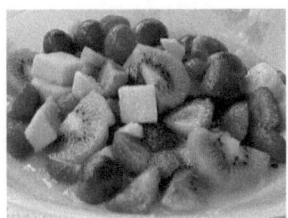

Enjoy this healthy Mediterranean-inspired version of the classic fruit salad.

Ingredients

- 1 lb. strawberries (quartered)
- ½ lb. blueberries
- ½ lb. blackberries
- ½ lb. raspberries
- Juice from 3 oranges
- Juice from 1 lemon
- 1 handful fresh mint (chopped)

Method

1. In a large bowl, mix berries together. Add orange and lemon juice. Stir to coat. Cover and chill 2 hours.

21. Macaroon Ice Cream Cake

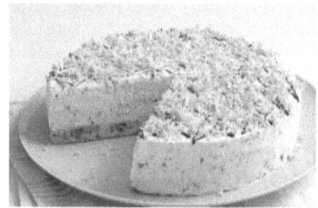

This coconut-chocolate treat is a sweet way to cool off this summer.

Ingredients

- 2 pints chocolate ice cream
- 2 pints vanilla almond ice cream
- 1 package soft coconut macaroons
- ½ cup chocolate shell ice cream topping
- 1 cup sliced almonds

Method

1. Lightly grease a baking dish (8"x3") with butter. Crumble half of the macaroons. Spread across the bottom of the dish (and about 1" up the sides). Spread a layer of chocolate ice cream evenly on top of macaroon crust.

2. Crumble remaining macaroons. Spread evenly over chocolate ice cream. Freeze 45 minutes. Spread a layer of vanilla almond ice cream

on top. Let freeze 4 hours. Pour chocolate topping on top of cake. Tilt dish to spread coating across the top. Let harden. Wrap a damp, warm towel around pan to loosen sides. Remove cake. Press sliced almonds onto the sides.

22. Chocolate Muffin Sandwiches

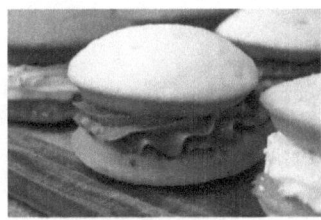

Chocolate muffins and ice cream combine for a simple and delicious dessert.

Ingredients

- 1 cup (+ 6 tbsp.) vanilla ice cream
- 4 chocolate chip muffins
- 4 large strawberries (sliced)

Method

1. Use a small ice cream scoop to scoop out 4 ice cream balls. Set on plate and store in freezer. Cut muffins in half horizontally. Press a small indentation in the cut side of the bottom piece with a spoon. Melt 1 cup ice cream in a small pot over low heat, stirring often.

2. Place one ball ice cream in each indent made in the muffin bottoms. Place the muffin top on and spoon over with melted ice cream. Sprinkle with strawberries.

23. Ginger Peach Ice Cream Pie

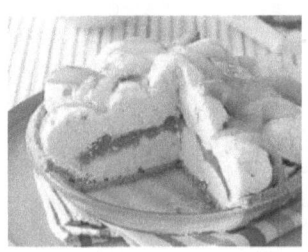

This pie recipe is light and refreshing—perfect for a hot summer day.

Ingredients

- 12 cinnamon graham crackers (crumbled)
- 5 tbsp. butter
- 1/3 cup chopped crystallized ginger
- 1 ½ cups peach preserves
- 8 cups peach ice cream
- 1 peach (thinly sliced)

Method

1. Lightly grease a 9" pie dish. Mix together graham cracker crumbs, butter, and 2 tablespoons ginger until combined. Spread crumb mixture in an even layer across bottom and sides of dish. Freeze for 30 minutes. Stir together peach preserves and remaining ginger.

2. Scoop 4 cups ice cream into pie dish. Place scoops close together. Do not spread. Pour 1 cup peach mixture over the top. Scoop in remaining ice cream. Freeze 3 hours. Stir fresh peach slices into remaining peach mixture. Cover and chill. Spoon peach mixture on top of pie before serving.

24. Raspberry-Orange Sherbet Cake

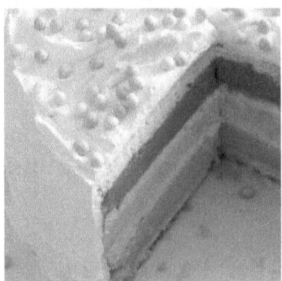

Raspberry and orange ice cream gives this cake a sweet and tangy touch.

Ingredients

- 2 packages coconut macaroons
- 3 cups raspberry sherbet
- 2 pints vanilla ice cream
- 3 cups orange sherbet

- 1 orange (peeled, sliced)
- 2 cups raspberries
- ½ cup water
- ½ cup sugar

Method

1. In a pot over medium-high heat, stir together water and sugar until dissolved. Stir in orange slices and raspberries. Bring to a boil. Let cook for 10 minutes. Remove from heat. Set aside.

2. Line a baking dish (13"x9") with foil. Allow 2" foil to hang over each short side. Lightly grease with butter. Arrange a layer of macaroons on the bottom of the dish. Drop in spoonfuls of sherbet and ice cream. Alternate flavors and pack down as you go until the bottom is covered.

3. Spread a layer of fruit mixture over the top. Freeze for 2 hours. Add remaining sherbet and ice cream in spoonfuls. Freeze for 30 minutes. Add remaining fruit mixture and another layer of macaroons. Freeze for 6 hours.

25. Lemon Ices

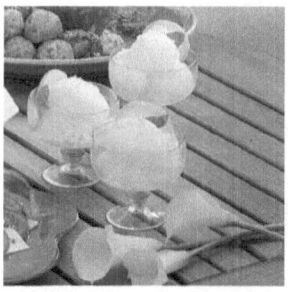

This chilly and zesty beverage is the perfect thing to sip when you're lounging poolside.

Ingredients

- Zest from 1 lemon
- Juice from 2 lemons
- 1 cup sugar
- 4 cups milk

Method

1. In a bowl, combine lemon zest, lemon juice, and sugar. Stir well, and then add milk. Pour into a 9"x9" dish and freeze. Let chill for 2 hours (stir once after 1 hour). Crush and pour into glasses.

26. Mango Sorbet

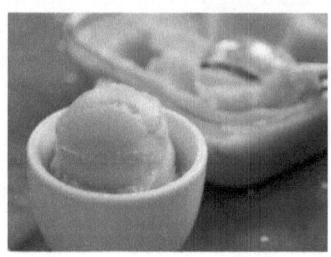

Make your own tropical sorbet with this simple recipe.

Ingredients

- 4 mangoes (cubed)
- 1 cup water
- 1 cup sugar
- 3 tbsp. fresh lime juice
- Ice cream maker

Method

1. In a small pot over medium-high heat, stir water and sugar until dissolved. Remove from heat. Puree mango in a food processor. Add sugar mixture and lime juice. Pulse until combined. Place mixture into an ice cream maker and prepare according to directions.

27. Ice Cream Snow

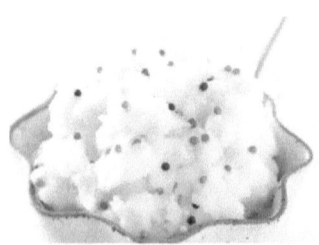

Stock up on fresh snow throughout the winter to make this delectable dessert come summer time!

Ingredients

- 1-gallon fresh snow or shaved ice
- 1 cup sugar
- 2 cups milk
- 1 tbsp. vanilla extract

Method

1. Stir ingredients together in a large serving bowl until well combined. Serve immediately.

28. Lime Coconut Sorbet

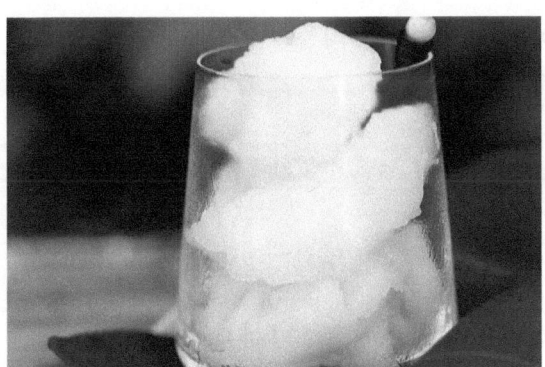

Lime gives this tropical sorbet a perfect hint of tanginess.

Ingredients

- 1 (15oz.) can coconut cream
- ¾ cup water
- ½ cup fresh lime juice
- Ice cream maker

Method

1. Mix ingredients together in an ice cream maker. Prepare according to directions.

29. Creamy Avocado Pops

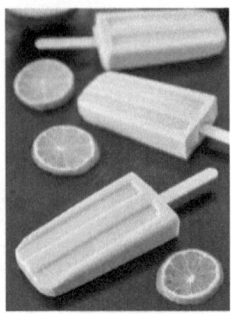

Avocado provides a rich creaminess and unique flavor to these summery treats.

Ingredients

- 3 avocados (peeled, pitted)
- 1 cup water
- ½ cup sugar
- Juice from 1 lime
- ¼ tsp salt

Method

1. In a small pot, bring water and sugar to a boil. Stir constantly until dissolved. Remove from heat. Let cool. In a blender, pulse everything together until smooth. Pour mixture into Popsicle molds. Freeze 2 hours. Insert sticks. Freeze overnight.

30. Chocolate Almond Bars

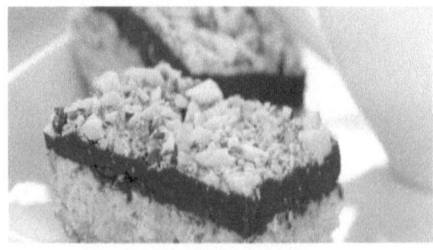

This ice-cream bar recipe can be varied to suit your taste with any flavor of ice cream or by substituting peanuts for almonds.

Ingredients

- 1 cup almonds (toasted)
- ½ gallon coffee or vanilla-flavored ice cream
- 2 pounds semi-sweet chocolate (chopped)
- 3 tbsp. solid vegetable shortening
- 12 flat wooden sticks

Method

1. Cut the block of ice cream into thirds. Set aside two-thirds and place in freezer. Cut the remaining block into 8 equal slices, about ½-inch thick. Using a spatula, transfer 4 pieces of ice cream to parchment paper lined baking sheet. Gently press each wooden stick lengthwise onto half of each piece. Top each piece with another ice cream piece to form a bar.

2. Cover with parchment paper or plastic wrap. Place baking sheet in freezer for about an hour or until it is firm. Repeat with remaining two-thirds of ice cream block. Place the finely chopped almonds in a shallow pie plate or dish. With a spatula, lift bars into dish and press the chopped nuts onto the sides and edges.

3. Cover the bars with plastic wrap and freeze for about 2 hours. Combine chocolate and shortening. Place in microwave for 2 minutes. Stir until the chocolate is completely melted. If chocolate is not completely melted, microwave 30 to 60 seconds more, then stir the mixture again.

4. Remove wrap from ice cream bars. Quickly dip a bar in the chocolate mixture using a spoon or rubber spatula. Return bars to freezer after dipping them. Chocolate should harden almost immediately. Freeze for 2 hours. Serve.

31. Fresh-Fruit Popsicles

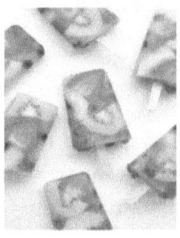

These fresh-fruit popsicles are the best treats to beat the summer heat.

Ingredients

- 2 cups fruit punch
- ½ cup raspberries
- ½ cup blueberries
- 2 kiwis (peeled and sliced into ¼-inch rounds)
- 1 peach (sliced)
- ¾ cup strawberries (finely chopped)

Method

1. Mix all the fruits in a bowl. Arrange the mixture into 8 3-ounce popsicle molds. Pour enough juice to cover the fruits in each mold. Insert popsicle sticks. Freeze for about 6 hours or until solid.

32. Peanut Butter Cookie Dough Bars

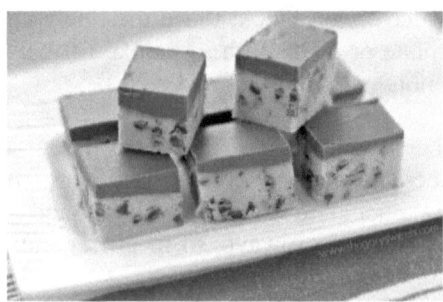

These cookie dough bars will give a fun twist to your peanut butter snack.

Ingredients

- ¼ cup creamy peanut butter
- ½ cup unsalted butter (softened)
- ¾ cup light brown sugar (packed)
- 1 tbsp. pure vanilla extract
- 2 cups all-purpose flour
- 14 oz. sweetened condensed milk
- 2 cups mini chocolate chip morsels
- ¾ cup creamy peanut butter (for frosting)
- ¾ cup semi-sweet chocolate chip morsels

Method

1. Beat softened butter with brown sugar until fully combined. Add vanilla and peanut butter, beat until fluffy. Add flour and sweetened condensed milk. Beat until everything is blended well. Fold in the mini chocolate chip morsels. Press into a baking dish (8"x8").

2. In a microwave safe, medium sized bowl, add peanut butter and chocolate chips for the frosting. Melt for one minute. Stir and spread over the cookie dough. Refrigerate for 3 hours or overnight. Cut into bite sized pieces and serve. You may store this snack in a covered container for up to a week.

33. Cookies and Cream Melt-Aways

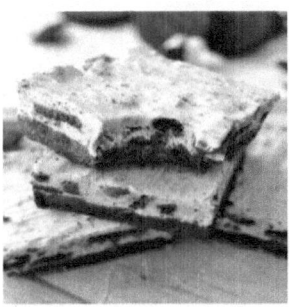

This no-bake treat is so easy even kids can make it.

Ingredients

- 40 Oreos (divided)
- 1 cup unsalted butter
- 3 cups powdered sugar
- 2 tbsp. milk
- 1 tsp. vanilla

Method

1. Finely crush 30 Oreos. You may use a food processor to make it easier. Combine the Oreo crumbs with softened butter. Press it into a pan (9"x9") to form a crust. Chill crust until firm.

2. Mix powdered sugar, softened butter, milk, and vanilla in a medium mixing bowl. Blend in medium-high speed for 2-3 minutes. Crush

remaining 10 Oreos, leaving some larger pieces. Stir into powdered sugar mixture. Spread mixture over top of crust and keep refrigerated until ready to serve.

34. Orange Cream Freezer Dessert

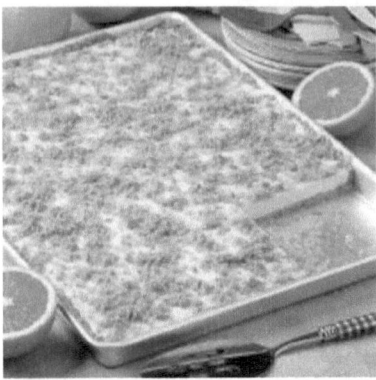

This dessert will please a crowd with its bold orange taste and cool smooth texture.

Ingredients

- 1 cup butter (Melted)
- ¾ cups sugar
- 3 ½ quarts vanilla ice cream (softened)
- 4 cups graham cracker crumbs
- 24 oz. orange juice concentrate (thawed from freezer)

Method

1. Combine sugar and graham cracker crumbs in a large bowl. Add in melted butter. Put aside about 2 cups for topping use later. As for the remaining crumb mixture, press them into two greased pans (15" x 10" x 1"). Cover and place in the freezer for about 15 minutes.

2. Blend the orange juice concentrate and ice cream until mixture is smooth. Spoon over the crusts and allow to freeze for 10 minutes or until the texture is a little firm. Sprinkle the reserved crumb mixture on top of orange juice and ice cream mixture then softly press down. Cover and let it freeze. Remove from freezer about 15 minutes right before serving.

35. Ice Cream Sandwich Cake

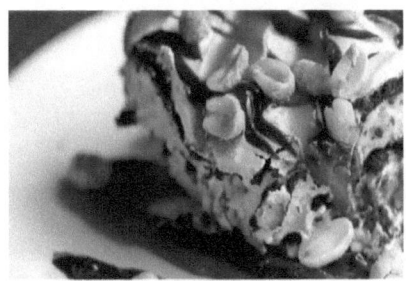

This recipe will give a sumptuous homemade taste to the usual store-bought ice cream sandwich.

Ingredients

- 16 Oz. Cool Whip
- 24 Ice Cream Sandwiches
- 1 Jar Caramel Sundae Topping
- 1 Bag of Reese's Peanut Butter Cups (coarsely chopped)

Method

1. Place half of the ice cream sandwiches in a pan (9" x 13"). Cover the sandwiches with half of the Cool Whip plus half of the caramel sundae topping and half of the Reese's cups.

2. Place the remaining ice cream sandwiches on top in the form of a top layer. Toss up with the left Cool Whip and distribute the whip evenly using a spatula. Top it with the remaining Reese's cups. Place the pan in the freezer for a few hours before serving.

36. Pink Lemonade Pie

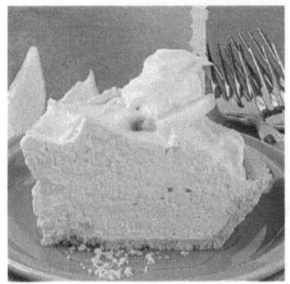

The luscious color of this treat will make any summer day more vibrant and fun.

Ingredients

- 2 and ½ Cups Graham Cracker Crumbs
- ½ Cup Sugar
- 10 Tbsps. Butter (melted)
- 3/4 of 12 oz. Canned Pink Lemonade (thawed)
- 16 oz. Cool Whip
- 1 Can Sweetened Condensed Milk
- Pink Food Coloring

Method

1. To make the crust, mix the cracker crumbs, sugar, and butter. Pour the mixture into a baking pan. Press it into the bottom of a pie dish by using a large spoon. Bake at 350 degrees for 8 minutes. Set aside. Pour condense milk as well as pink lemonade in a bowl. Mix thoroughly. Add a few drops of food coloring until you get your desired shade of pink. Add more drops for a deeper pink hue. Mix in about 10 oz. of Cool Whip.

2. Whip up the pink lemonade concoction some more using a hand mixer. Pour the concoction into the crust. Allow it to set in the fridge for several hours then top it with the remaining Cool Whip. Let it chill in the freezer for a few hours before serving.

37. Layered Melon Kiwi Jell-O Cups

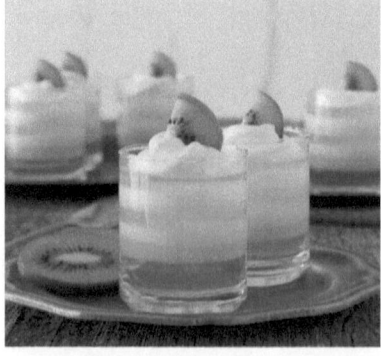

This five-layered dessert will surely make summer awesome.

Ingredients

- 5 Packs of Melon Fusion Jell-O Mix
- 2 and ½ cups Cool Whip
- 6 to 8 Kiwi (sliced)
- 5 Cups Water (boiled)

Method

1. Add boiled water with one pack of Jell-O mix. Stir until the Jell-O has fully dissolved. Add a cup of cold water to the mixture and stir some more. Place the mixture into molding cups and refrigerate for 1 hour. To make the second layer, repeat steps by mixing a cup of boiled water to a pack of Jell-O mix. Add a cup of cool whip and stir until mixed well. Put on top of the first layer. Set in the fridge for an hour.

2. For the third layer, repeat the procedure for the first layer. Again, refrigerate for another hour. To make the fourth and final layers, repeat step. This time, allow the mixture to set in the fridge for two hours. Top the final layer with a spoonful of Cool Whip and kiwi slices. Serve.

38. Banana Split Fluff Salad

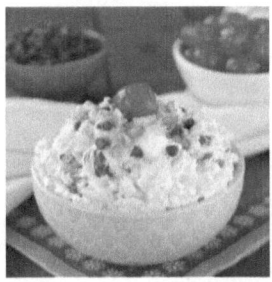

The fruits, nuts, and marshmallows give this salad a very interesting twist.

Ingredients

- 3.4 Oz. Instant Banana Pudding
- ½ Cup Mini Chocolate Chips
- 2 Ripe Bananas (sliced)
- 10 Oz. Jar Maraschino Cherries (halved)
- 20 Oz. Can Crushed Pineapple (not drained)
- 8 Oz. Cool Whip

- 1 Cup Mini Marshmallows
- ½ Cup Walnuts (finely chopped)
- 2 Tbsps. Walnuts (chopped and to be used as garnish)

Method

1. Combine the pudding mix and pineapple thoroughly. Fold in the Cool Whip. Gradually add the marshmallows, chocolate chips, bananas, cherries and nuts. Leave mixture in the fridge for about an hour prior to serving.

39. Raspberry Sorbet

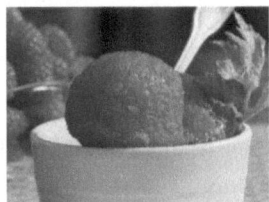

This creamy treat provides a perfect way to cool down this summer.

Ingredients

- 5 Cups Raspberries (fresh)
- 1 ½ Cup Sugar
- 1 Tsp. Vanilla Extract
- 1 - 2 Tbsps. Fresh Lemon Juice
- 1 Cup Water

Method

1. Add water to the raspberries and mix using a food processor in Pulse mode. Continue pulsing until mixture is fully blended. Using a fine mesh strainer placed over a large bowl sieve the pureed raspberries. Do so by adding ¼ of the raspberries at a time.

2. The next step involves removing the berries' seeds. Do so by pressing a large spoon or a rubber spatula against the raspberry puree through a strainer. Discard what's left in the strainer.

3. In a large bowl, combine the sugar, vanilla, and lemon juice and mix in the raspberry juice. Beat until the sugar has completely dissolved.

Freeze for an hour. You may also serve instantly if you want a soft-serve treat.

40. Banana Chocolate Ice Cream

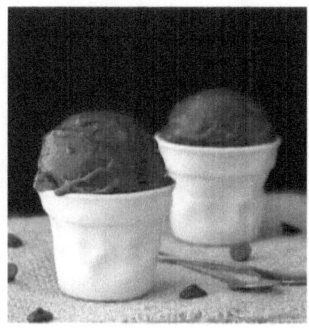

This frozen treat is very easy to make with its two ingredients.

Ingredients

- 2 Tbsps. Cocoa Powder
- 3 Bananas (sliced and frozen)

Method

1. Take the frozen bananas and turn them into puree using a blender or food processor. Keep on blending until mixture is smooth and creamy. Add the cocoa powder to the banana puree. Mix until you get the thickness of a soft-served ice cream. Keep cold in the freezer for up to two hours before serving.

41. Cherry Vanilla Coca-Cola Ice Cream Float

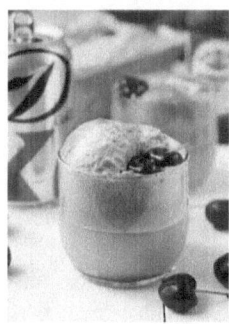

This classic beverage brings out the best in vanilla ice cream for one ultimate refreshing summer dessert recipe.

Ingredients

- 6 Cups Coca-Cola
- 2 Cups Vanilla Ice Cream
- 4 Tbsps. Cherry Syrup

Method

1. Take 4 drinking glasses and place half a cup of ice cream in each glass. Pour cola close to the brim of each glass and watch it foam. Add a tablespoon of cherry syrup per glass. You can add more depending on your preference. Stir and serve.

42. Chocolate Cake Ice Cream Truffles

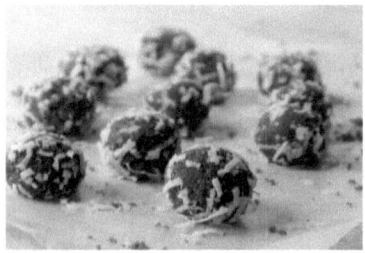

These bite-sized treats take ice cream and cake crumbs to form a perfect delectable pair.

Ingredients

- 2 Cups Chocolate Cake Crumbs
- 1 Scoop Vanilla Ice Cream (melted)
- 1 ½ Cups Shredded Coconut

Method

1. Use a wax paper to line a plate then set aside. Put the cake crumbs in a medium-size mixing bowl. Pour melted ice cream over the cake crumbs. Mix well. Form 2-inch balls using the cake-ice cream mixture. Roll and coat each ball on shredded coconut. Place cookies in the freezer for 30 minutes or until firm. Serve.

43. Frozen Grasshopper Squares

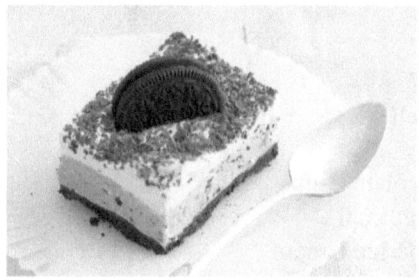

This simple and easy four-ingredient frozen dessert for summer will leave you refreshed yet wanting more.

Ingredients

- 28 Oreo Cookies (divided)
- 8 Oz. Cool Whip (thawed)
- 1 Oz. Semi-Sweet Chocolate (grated)
- 6 Cups Chocolate Chip Mint Ice Cream (softened)

Method

1. Line a pan (13" x 9") with aluminum foil. Crush 20 cookies and sprinkle onto bottom of pan. Spread ice cream over the crumbs in pan and top with a layer of Cool whip plus grated chocolate. Refrigerate for 3 hours. Remove from freezer 15 minutes before serving. Cut remaining cookies in half and use them to garnish the dessert squares.

44. Ice Cream Sundae Cookie Cups

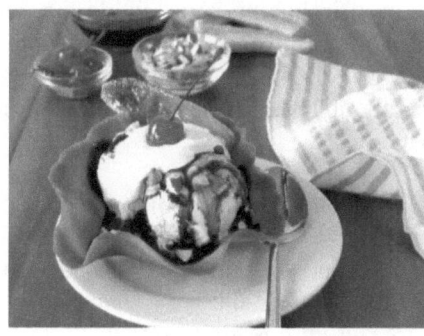

The different textures and rich taste of this amazing treat will keep you refreshed and fully satisfied.

Ingredients

For the chocolate shell

- 1/2 Cup Chocolate Chips
- 3 Tsps. Coconut Oil
- 3 Cups Vanilla Ice Cream
- 1/4 Cup Peanuts (chopped)

For the cookie cups

- 1 Stick Softened Butter
- ½ Cup Brown Sugar
- ½ Cup Sugar
- 1 Egg
- 1 Tsp. Vanilla
- 1 ½ Cup All-Purpose Flour
- 1/4 teaspoon salt
- 1/2 Tsp. Baking Soda

Method

1. Preheat oven to 350 degrees. Cream together butter, sugar and brown sugar. Add egg and vanilla to the butter-sugar mixture until smooth and creamy. Mix flour, salt and baking soda in a separate bowl. Slowly add the dry ingredients to the batter.

2. Use an ice cream scooper to scoop dough onto a greased standard sized 12-piece muffin baking pan. Divide the dough evenly between the 12 cups. Bake for 15 minutes. Remove from oven and press down the center of each cookie using a small spice container. Let cool for 10 minutes. Place about 1/4 cup vanilla ice cream on top of each cookie cup. Refrigerate.

3. To create the chocolate shell, combine coconut oil and the chocolate chips in a small microwavable bowl. Microwave for 20 seconds. Remove from oven and stir until the chips have fully dissolved. Spoon the chocolate mixture over the ice cream and sprinkle with peanuts. Return to the freezer until ready to serve.

45. Pineapple Coconut Frozen Yogurt

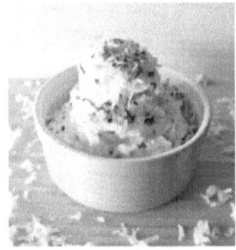

The pineapple and coconut in this recipe creates a fun light dessert that will bring out smiles on any hot day.

Ingredients

- ½ Cup Plain Greek Yogurt
- 1 Tbsp. Vodka
- ¼ Cup Pineapple (crushed and drained)
- ¾ Cup Reduced-Fat Coconut Milk
- 6 Tbsps. Granulated Sugar

Method

1. Combine the yogurt, coconut milk, sugar and vodka in a blender. Pulse until mixed thoroughly. Cover and place in the refrigerator for at least 2 hours. Pour the yogurt mixture into an ice cream maker. Process according to the manufacturer's directions.

2. Transfer the frozen yogurt to a large container with a lid and stir in the crushed pineapple. Mix well to avoid any pineapple juice ice chunks. Cover and place back into the freezer until solid. Serve.

46. Hazelnut Mocha Ice Cream

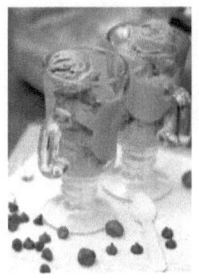

This high-protein and sugar-free dessert is a healthy way to beat the summer heat.

Ingredients

- 32 Oz. Plain and Nonfat Greek Yogurt
- 1 Cup Healthy Homemade Nutella
- 1 Tbsp. Vanilla-Flavored Stevia Extract
- 1/8 Tsp. Pink Himalayan Salt
- 1 Tsp. Xanthan Gum
- 2/3 Cup Espresso

Method

1. Take an ice cream maker bowl and freeze it overnight. Whisk together the yogurt, salt, espresso, Nutella and stevia extract. You may also use an electric mixer set to the low speed setting.

2. Continue to whisk the yogurt mixture by hand or increase the mixer's speed to medium. Gradually add the Xanthan gum. With a rubber spatula, scrape the sides of the bowl. Take a whisk and with it combine the batter until it has a thick and even consistency. Cover the bowl and leave in the fridge overnight.

3. Take the frozen ice cream maker bowl and place it on a stand mixer. Set it to the "stir" speed. Scoop out the ice cream mixture from the spinning bowl. Churn the ice cream until you achieve a soft-serve quality. Leave mixture in the fridge just before serving.

47. Layered Berry Vanilla Soft Serve

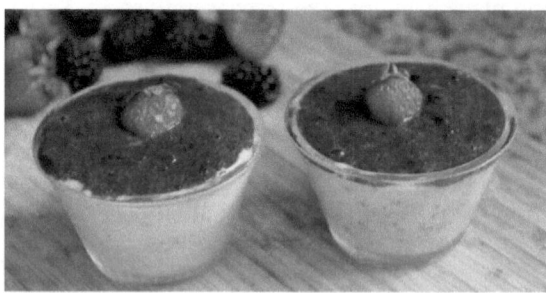

Incorporating fruit in this frozen treat gives this dish an extra serving of freshness this summer.

Ingredients

- 4 Medium-Sized Bananas
- ½ Cup Strawberries (either frozen or fresh)
- ½ Cup Blackberries (either frozen or fresh)
- ¼ Tsp. Vanilla Extract

Method

1. Chop the bananas and place each banana in its own re-sealable plastic bag. Freeze overnight. Remove bananas from the freezer and thaw for 15 minutes. Using a food processor, blend the banana pieces from one bag.

2. Add in vanilla extract and 1/3 cup water. Combine with the banana until mixture is smooth and thick. Scoop an equal amount of the banana puree mixture into the bottom of three separate serving dishes. Clean the food processor container before moving on to the next step.

3. For the next layer, add another bag of frozen banana pieces to the strawberries. Mix in a food processor until smooth. Distribute the mixture evenly among the three separate serving dishes containing the first layer of bananas you previously created. You now have the second layer.

4. Clean the food processor container once more. For the last layer, add the blueberries and blackberries to the food processor. If the blueberries are frozen, add 1/4 cup of water. Blend until smooth. Distribute the berry mixture evenly among the three separate serving dishes once more. You now have the top and final layer. Serve immediately.

48. Snickerdoodle Ice Cream Sandwiches

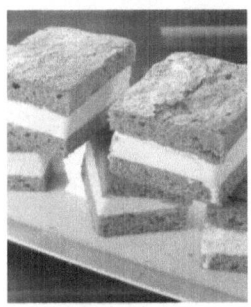

This special dessert is made up of only three simple ingredients yet you're left with a snack to crave on any hot summer day.

Ingredients

For the sugar cookies

- ¾ Cups All-Purpose Flour
- ¼ Tsp. Fine Sea Salt
- 1 Stick Unsalted Butter
- 2 Oz. Cream Cheese
- ¾ Cup Granulated White Sugar
- ½ Tsp. Baking Powder
- ¼ Tsp. Baking Soda
- 1 Egg (large)
- 1 Tsp. Vanilla Extract
- ¼ Cup Granulated White Sugar (combined with ½ Tsp. Ground Cinnamon)

For the cinnamon ice cream

- 1 ½ Cup Whole Milk
- 2 Tsps. Ground Cinnamon
- 1 Tsp. Vanilla Extract
- 4 Egg Yolks (large)
- 1 ½ Cup Heavy Cream
- 3/4 Cup Granulated White Sugar
- 1/4 Tsp. Fine Sea Salt

Method

1. To make the ice cream, prepare an ice bath by filling a large bowl with ice cubes and 1 to 2 cups of water. Place a medium bowl fitted with a fine strainer inside the ice bath. Combine the milk, cream, 1/2 cup sugar, salt, cinnamon and vanilla. Set over medium heat, making sure to stir occasionally until the mixture is warm.

2. In a medium bowl, whisk together the egg yolks and remaining sugar. Whisk half of the warm milk mixture into the egg yolks. Whisk the egg-milk mixture back into the saucepan.

3. Cook the mixture over medium heat, stirring constantly with a wooden spoon. Immediately pour the mixture through the strainer into the bowl set over the ice bath. Let it cool in the ice bath until it reaches room temperature. Press plastic wrap against the surface of the custard and refrigerate until well chilled. Pour the chilled mixture into the bowl of your ice cream maker.

4. To make the cookies, line two large baking sheets with parchment paper. Whisk together the flour, baking powder, baking soda and salt to combine thoroughly. Use an electric mixer to beat the butter, cream cheese and 3/4 cup sugar on medium to high speed. Mix until smooth.

5. Add the egg and vanilla and beat on low speed. Slowly add the flour mixture and mix until combined well. Place the sugar-cinnamon mixture in a small bowl. Roll the dough into 2 tbsps.-sized balls and then roll the balls on sugar, making sure each ball is coated evenly. Place the dough balls on the prepared baking sheets.

6. Bake in oven for 10 to 12 minutes. Let the cookies cool for 5 minutes before transferring them onto a wire rack to cool fully. Freeze the cookies until firm. Place a scoop of ice cream on top of each cookie. Form a sandwich by placing another cookie on top of the ice cream and gently press down. Freeze for at least 2 hours before serving.

49. Lime Creamsicles

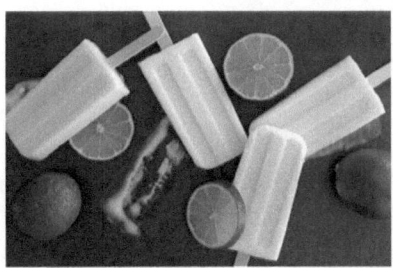

This simple and refreshing dessert will bring back memories of the best summer afternoons.

Ingredients

- ½ Cup Lime Juice (fresh)
- 14 Oz. Can Sweetened Condensed Milk
- 2 Cups Milk

Method

1. Combine the milk, lime juice and sweetened condensed milk in a large bowl. Pour the milk mixture into Popsicle molds. Place a Popsicle stick in the center of each mold. Cover and freeze overnight. Dip the mold in a bowl or container of warm water for 15 seconds to easily remove popsicles from the mold. Serve.

50. Greek Yogurt Fudgesicles

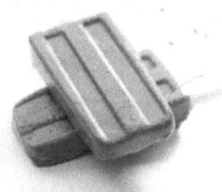

These creamy fudgesicles are the perfect treats on warm days with the ones you love.

Ingredients

- 1 Cup Plain Non-Fat Greek Yogurt
- ½ Cup Unsweetened Cocoa
- 2/3 Cup Agave Nectar
- 1 Cup Skim Milk
- 2 Tbsps. Vanilla Extract

Method

1. Mix all of the ingredients in a blender. Blend until smooth. Pour the mixture into Popsicle molds. Freeze for at least 4 hours. Serve.

51. Chocolate-Dipped Pear Popsicles

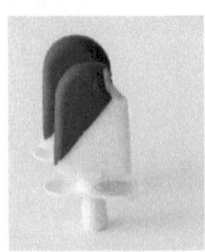

These fruit popsicles are easy to make and will leave everyone refreshed and wishing for more.

Ingredients

- 2 Pears (peeled, cored and sliced)
- ½ Cup Water
- ⅛ Cup Simple Syrup
- 1 Tbsp. Lemon Juice (fresh)

For the chocolate coating

- 1 Cup Dark Chocolate Chips
- 2 Tbsps. Coconut Oil

Method

1. Combine the pears, water, simple syrup and fresh lemon juice in a blender or food processor. Puree until smooth. Fill up Popsicle molds with the puree. Freeze for an hour.

2. To make the coating, combine the chocolate chips and coconut oil in a microwave-safe bowl. Microwave for around 30 seconds. The chocolate chips should be soft. Remove the mixture from the microwave and stir together until smooth. Cool slightly. Once popsicles are frozen, pull them out from the molds and quickly dip into the chocolate mixture.

52. Salted Caramel Milkshake

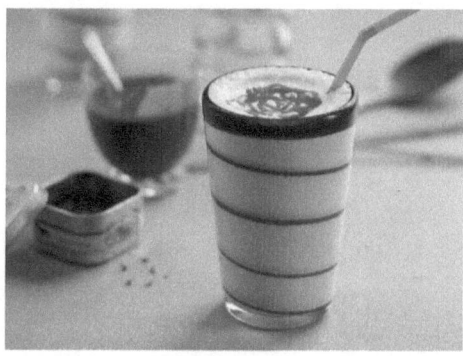

This milkshake recipe will make every summer day a day to look forward to.

Ingredients

- 2 Cups Vanilla Bean Ice Cream (packed)
- ½ Cup Milk
- 3 Tbsps. Salted Caramel Syrup
- 4 Ghirardelli Dark Chocolate and Sea Salt Caramel Squares

Method

1. Using an electric blender, combine the ice cream, milk, caramel syrup and Ghirardelli Dark Chocolate and Sea Salt Caramel Squares on medium to high speed. Blend until thoroughly combined. Top off the milkshake with whipped cream, caramel sauce and chocolate sprinkles (optional). Serve right away.

53. Coconut Granita

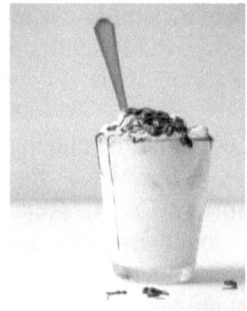

This exotic dessert is so delicious you'll vow to have it in your freezer all summer long.

Ingredients

- 14 Oz. Full-Fat Coconut Milk
- ¼ Cup Honey
- ¼ Cup Water
- Half a Lime (optional)
- Chocolate Sauce (optional)

Method

1. Pour the coconut milk in a shallow dish. Combine the sugar and water in a small microwave-safe dish. Microwave until the water simmers.

Remove from oven and stir to dissolve the sugar. Let cool slightly then add to the coconut milk.

2. Squeeze lime juice into mixture if you desire. Place the mixture in the freezer, scraping it every 30 minutes for up to 2 hours. Serve with chocolate sauce drizzled on top.

54. Chocolate Frosting Shots

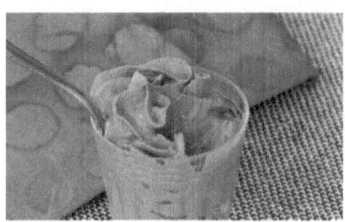

This healthy frosting recipe is a super fun way to beat the summer heat.

Ingredients

- 1 Can Full-Fat Coconut Milk
- ¼ Cup plus 1 Tbsp. Cocoa Powder
- ½ Tsp. Pure Vanilla Extract
- Powdered Sugar (for thickening)

Method

1. Thicken coconut milk by leaving the can uncovered in the fridge overnight. Once thick, transfer only the creamy part to a bowl, leaving the watery part out. Whip in cocoa, vanilla and sweetener using a fork. Pipe the chocolate frosting shots out using an icing tip. Set in the fridge for an hour before serving.

55. Strawberry Crème Truffles

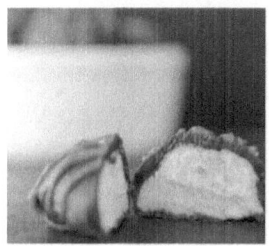

This melt-in-the-mouth goodness is very easy to make and will satisfy you sweet tooth like no other.

Ingredients

For the chocolate

- 1 Cup Dark Chocolate Chips
- 3 Tbsp. Almond Milk

For the filling

- 1 Cup Coconut Butter
- 1 Cup Strawberries (sliced)
- 2 Tbsp. Maple Syrup

Method

1. Mix the ingredients for the filling using a food processor. Drop small balls of the filling onto a lined baking sheet using a cookie scoop. Let it chill for 15 minutes.

2. Stick the baking sheet containing all the coconut balls in the freezer to stiffen. Melt the chocolate chips and the milk using a double boiler. Stir constantly until all the chips are melted and the mixture is smooth. Use two forks to roll the balls into the chocolate. Place them back onto the lined baking sheet. Stick the balls back into the freezer for about 30 minutes to 1 hour. Serve.

56. Frozen Cookie Dough Bites

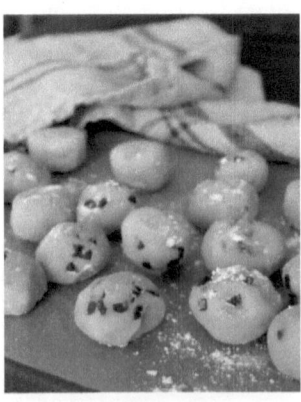

This delicious cookie dough is so mouthwatering you will wish everyday was a warm sunny day for extra reasons.

Ingredients

- 4 Oz. Butter (unsalted and set to room temperature)
- 1 Tsp. Vanilla Extract
- 6 ½ Oz. Flour
- 1 Tsp. Cinnamon
- 1 Tsp. Salt
- 3 Oz. Granulated Sugar
- 3 Oz. Brown Sugar
- 4-6 Oz. Chocolate Chips

Method

1. Mix the sugar, vanilla extract and butter until consistency is fluffy. Add in the flour, salt and cinnamon. Blend together until a dough-like texture is achieved.

2. Add the chocolate chips and blend until evenly spread all over. Take the dough and roll it into small bowls. Place dough on lined baking sheet. Pop in the dough into the freezer and leave it there for about 20 to 25 minutes. Remove from freezer when dough is solid and firm. Serve.

57. S'mores Ice Cream Sandwiches

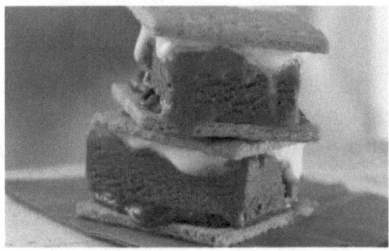

This chocolate-dipped dessert is such a masterpiece and is sure to be a big hit at any party.

Ingredients

- ¼ Cup All-Purpose Flour
- 1 Tbsp. Cornstarch

- ¼ Cup Light Brown Sugar
- 2 Tbsps. Granulated Sugar
- 1 Tbsp. Honey
- ½ Tsp. Vanilla Extract
- 2 Tbsps. Whole Milk
- ½ Tsp. Baking Soda
- ½ Tsp. Salt
- ¾ Stick Butter (unsalted)

For the sandwich

- 1 Batch of Toasted Marshmallow Ice Cream
- 1/3 Cup Marshmallow Topping
- 8 Oz. Semi-Sweet Chocolate (finely chopped)

Method

1. Evenly spread out churned ice cream onto a baking pan lined with parchment paper. Cover with plastic wrap and freeze overnight. To make the cookies, preheat the oven to 350-degree F. Line two baking sheets with parchment paper. Whisk together the flour, cornstarch, baking soda and salt. Set aside in a bowl.

2. In another bowl, beat butter on medium-high speed for 1 to 2 minutes. Add sugars, honey and vanilla and beat until light and fluffy. Pour in half of the dry ingredients and mix on low speed until combined well, but not thoroughly. Add in milk and continue mixing. Pop in the other dry ingredients and mix until dough comes together.

3. Roll out dough with 1/4-inch thickness on a floured surface. Cut into 2 1/4-inch squares using a knife or pizza cutter. Transfer the squares onto the baking sheets, leaving about 1 inch of space between the cookies. Re-roll the scraps and cut again until no dough remains. Bake for 10 to 12 minutes. Pull out from oven and let cool on baking sheets then transfer into a plastic re-sealable bag. Freeze until ready to use.

4. Arrange half of the cookies onto a baking sheet. Pull out ice cream from refrigerator and lift out the whole chunk of frozen ice cream. Divide into 16 even squares.

5. Place a square of ice cream on each upside-down cookie then top with leftover cookies, pressing lightly. Return entire tray to the freezer and allow to set until completely frozen once again. Make a second baking

sheet by lining it with parchment paper. Refrigerate for at least 15 minutes, allowing it to completely chill.

6. Slightly thaw out the chocolate using a double boiler. Dip sandwiches halfway into the melted chocolate and place on the baking sheet in the freezer. Work quickly to avoid melting. Once chocolate is set, wrap each sandwich in foil or plastic wrap. Store in a re-sealable plastic bag for up to 2 months.

58. Sweet Potato Ice Cream

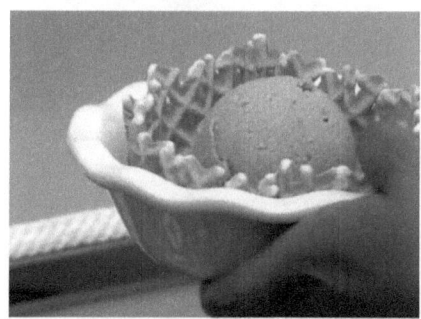

The sweet potato is a healthy alternative to sugar, especially when you're craving something sweet on a blistering summer day.

Ingredients

- Sweet potato (baked and peeled)
- 1 Tbsp. Maple Syrup
- 2 Tbsps. Cinnamon
- 1 Tsp. Vanilla Extract
- 1 Can Full-Fat Coconut Milk
- 2 Egg Yolks
- 1/8 Tsp. Nutmeg
- 1/8 Tsp. Sea Salt

Method

1. Place potato and coconut milk in a blender or food processor. Continue to blend until the thickness resembles that of puree. Add in cinnamon, vanilla extract, sea salt, nutmeg and egg yolks. Mix thoroughly. You may at times need to halt the food processor in order to scrape down the sides, in case the ingredients get stuck.

2. Pour mixture in a large bowl. Allow it to cool in the fridge for a minimum time of 2 hours. When mixture is set, use an ice cream maker to churn. Let it churn for about 30 minutes, or the time required by the ice cream maker's instruction. Once you got the thickness desired, remove it from the ice cream maker. Serve.

59. Raspberry Coconut Chia Ice Pops

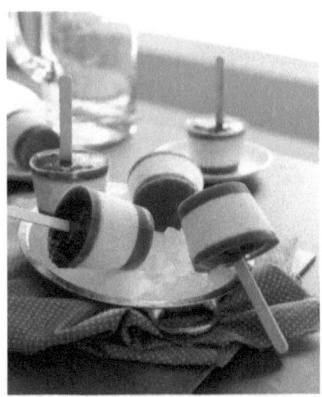

This recipe can be made with optional add-ins like honey, lime juice, coconut extract and vanilla extract for extra flair and fun.

Ingredients

- 15 Oz. Can Full-Fat Coconut Milk
- 1 ½ Tbsps. Chia Seeds
- 1 ½ Cup Raspberries (thawed)
- ½ Cup Water

Method

1. Place raspberries and water in a blender. Blend it until mixture is smooth. Add about 2 tablespoons of raspberry puree into a cup. Keep the leftover puree for later. Place cups in the chiller for half an hour.

2. Blend the coconut milk and Chia seeds in a small bowl. Remove the cups from the freezer. Add in the coconut mixture and return it to the freezer for another half an hour. Remove the cup and place a Popsicle stick upright in the middle. Place in the fridge for another 30 minutes. Add the extra raspberry puree and let it set for 3 hours. Strip the paper cups off before serving.

60. Caramel Candied Almonds

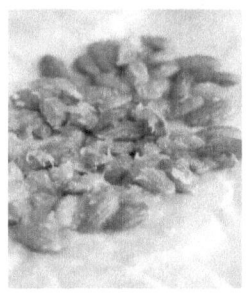

This simple dessert packs a high dose of vitamin E.

Ingredients

- 1 cup Almonds
- ½ cup Sugar
- 4 Tbsps. Butter
- ¼ tsp Vanilla Extract

Method

1. In a pan on medium-high heat, stir all ingredients together until sugar is dissolved and caramel-colored. Spread on a greased, lined baking sheet. Let cool completely. Break apart. Serve.

Health Benefits of Almonds

Rich source vitamin E which gives skin that youthful glow. High in phosphorus which strengthens bones and teeth. Speed up weight loss by improving digestion and controlling appetite.

61. Double Chocolate Chip Cookies

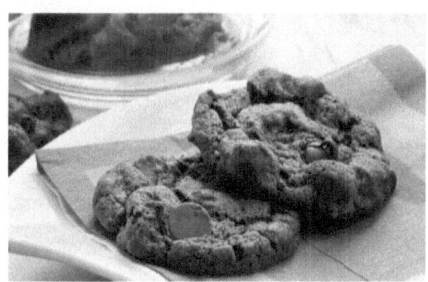

Indulge in luxurious chocolate with this cookie recipe.

Ingredients

- 4 cups Sugar
- 1 cup Butter
- 1 ½ cups Sugar
- 3 Tbsps. Molasses
- 2 large Eggs
- ¾ cup Cacao
- 2 Tbsps. Cornstarch
- 1 tsp Salt
- 2 cups Dark Chocolate Chunks

Method

1. In a bowl, combine butter and sugar until fluffy. Whisk in egg and molasses. In a separate bowl, combine flour, cacao, baking soda, cornstarch, and salt. Gradually add dry ingredients to wet ingredients. Blend until combined. Fold in chocolate chunks. Mix well. Separate dough into approximately 24 small balls. Freeze 2 hours. Place frozen dough balls on parchment lined baking sheet. Bake for 12-18 minutes at 350°F.

Health Benefits of Dark Chocolate (70% Cacao)

Improves circulation. Rich source of antioxidants. Lowers Cholesterol.

62. Frozen Chocolate Chip Cookie Dough Yogurt

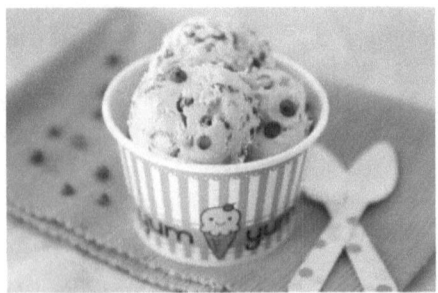

This recipe combines all the fun of eating cookie dough without the health risks!

Ingredients

- 6 oz. Greek Yogurt
- 1 Tbsp. Peanut or Almond Butter
- 1 Tbsp. Honey
- 2 Tbsps. Dark Chocolate Chunks
- ¼ tsp Vanilla Extract
- 1 pinch Salt

Method

1. Combine all ingredients in a bowl. Mix well. Freeze 1-2 hours. Serve.

Health Benefits of Greek Yogurt

Adds essential probiotics to your digestive system. Improves health of reproductive organs. Lowers blood pressure.

63. Nutella & Cream Popsicles

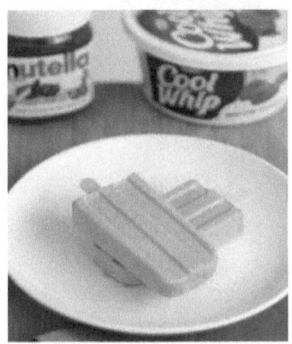

Make your own scrumptious popsicles with this simple recipe.

Ingredients

- 13 ½ oz. Coconut Milk
- 1 Egg
- 2 cups Nutella
- 1/3 cup Raw Hazelnuts (chopped)
- 2 tsp Vanilla Extract
- 2 Tbsps. Honey
- Paper cups & popsicle sticks

Method

1. In a pan on medium heat, whisk together coconut milk, egg, honey, and vanilla extract. Heat until bubbly. Refrigerate 4 hours (or overnight). Process in an ice cream maker according to instructions. Place a layer of the ice cream on the bottom of each paper cup.

2. Place a layer of chopped hazelnuts on top followed by a layer of Nutella. Repeat layering until cups are full. Push a Popsicle stick down in the middle. Freeze until set. Tear away paper cup. Serve.

Health Benefits of Hazelnuts

Lowers bad cholesterol. Helps your body absorb nutrients. High protein and magnesium help build muscle.

64. Banana Bread Brownies

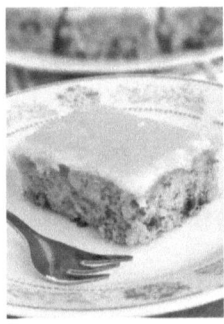

This recipe is a marriage between two dessert favorites: brownies and banana bread.

Ingredients

- 2 cups Whole Grain Flour
- 1 cup Sour Cream
- 1 cups Sugar
- 1 cup Powdered Sugar
- ½ cup Butter
- 1 ¾ cup Bananas (mashed)
- ¾ cup Peanut Butter
- 4 oz. Cream Cheese
- 2 Eggs
- 4 Tbsps. Milk

- 2 tsp Vanilla Extract
- 1 tsp Baking Soda
- ¾ tsp Salt

Method

1. Preheat oven to 375°F. In a bowl, beat together butter, sour cream, eggs, and sugar until smooth. Mix in vanilla extract and bananas. Add baking soda, salt, and flour. Beat until smooth. Pour into a greased ban. Bake 20 minutes. Remove. Let cool.

2. In a clean bowl, whisk together peanut butter and cream cheese until smooth. Whisk in milk and powdered sugar ½ cup at a time. Spread peanut butter frosting on top of cooled banana brownies.

Health Benefits of Bananas

Improves digestion. Stimulates the growth of friendly bacteria in your digestive track. Helps treat anemia.

65. Candied Blood Oranges

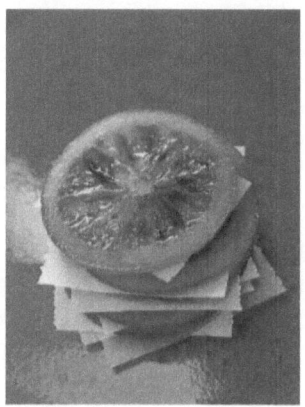

Try this delicious new way to enjoy your citrus.

Ingredients

- 1 cup Water
- 1 cup Sugar
- 1 Blood Orange

Method

1. With peel intact, cut blood orange into thin slices. In a large pan on medium-high heat, boil water and sugar. Stir until dissolved. Reduce heat to a simmer. Add orange slices. Cook 40 minutes. Turn slices every 10 minutes. Remove and arrange on a plate to cool.

Health Benefits of Blood Oranges

Rich in antioxidants that are missing from other citrus. High in folate. High in fiber.

66. Blackberry Cabernet Popsicles

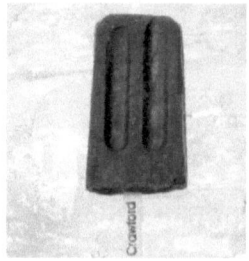

These popsicles are the perfect way to get your heart-healthy serving of red wine on a hot day!

Ingredients

- 2 cups Cabernet Sauvignon
- 1 cup Simple Syrup
- 1 cup Blackberries (chopped)
- Popsicle molds

Method

1. In a bowl or pitcher, mix cabernet and simple syrup. Distribute blackberries evenly among Popsicle molds. Fill molds with cabernet mixture. Freeze until set.

Health Benefits of Red Wine

Resveratrol in red wine helps lower bad cholesterol and prevent blood clots. Polyphenols help strengthen blood vessels. Lowers blood pressure.

67. Tangerine Prosecco Sorbet

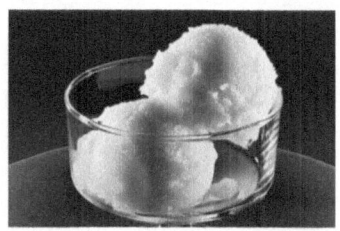

Prosecco and tangerine combine to create an unforgettable sorbet.

Ingredients

- ¾ cup Sugar
- ¾ cup Water
- 2 cups Chilled Tangerine Juice (from about 15 tangerines)
- 1 cup Chilled Prosecco
- 1 Tbsp. Tangerine Zest
- Ice Cream Maker

Method

1. In a small pan on medium heat, mix together water and sugar until sugar is dissolved. Increase heat and bring to a boil. Transfer to a bowl and chill 2 hours. Mix in prosecco, tangerine juice and zest. Blend well. Transfer to ice cream maker and process according to instructions. Transfer to a container and freeze 8 hours.

Health Benefits of Tangerine

Helps the body absorb iron. Lowers cholesterol. Improves digestion.

68. Candied Pumpkin and Yogurt Kataifi

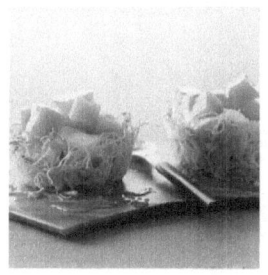

This dessert is wonderfully delicious and highly nutritious.

Ingredients

- 1 ½ cups Plain Greek Yogurt
- 1 cup Honey
- 2 cups Water
- 1/3 cup Sugar
- ¼ lbs. Kataifi (shredded phyllo dough)
- ½ cup Sliced Almonds
- 1 ¾ lbs. Pumpkin or Butternut Squash (peeled, seeded, cubed)
- 6 Tbsps. Butter (melted)
- 3 Tbsps. Powdered Sugar
- 3 Tbsps. Fresh Lemon Juice
- 1 Tbsp. Fresh Lemon Zest
- ½ tsp Cinnamon

Method

1. Place yogurt in a fine sieve lined with paper towels. Set over a bowl. Let drain 1 hour. Discard liquid. Preserve yogurt. Mix in 1 ½ tablespoons yogurt.

2. In a large pot over medium-high heat, boil water, sugar, cinnamon, 1 cup honey, lemon juice and zest. Stir until sugar is dissolved. Add pumpkin. Reduce heat, cover, and simmer 15-20 minutes. Remove pumpkin. Transfer to a bowl. Return syrup to a boil for 5-8 minutes. Preheat oven to 375°F.

3. In a bowl, whisk together powdered sugar and butter. Pull apart kataifi (the individual shredded pieces of pastry) and toss together with almonds and the butter mixture. Divide kataifi evenly into 12 muffin cups. Press into cups to create "nests". Bake 12-18 minutes. Let cool. Transfer kataifi to serving plates. Spoon in pumpkin. Drizzle over with syrup. Top with a dollop of yogurt.

Health Benefits of Pumpkin

Helps fight cravings and aid in weight loss. Improves sleep quality. Lowers blood pressure.

69. Honey Lemon Custard with Fruit

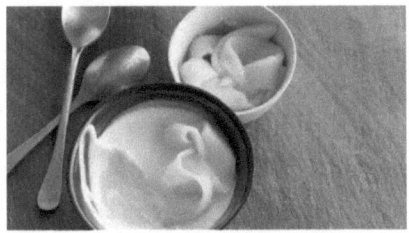

Finish off a dinner party with this bright and refreshing dessert.

Ingredients

- 2 cups Heavy Cream
- 1 cup Berries (or Sliced Mango)
- ¼ cup Light Rum
- 6 Tbsps. Fresh Lemon Juice (plus peel)
- 4 Tbsps. Honey
- 3 Tbsps. Sugar
- ½ vanilla bean (split lengthwise)

Method

1. Place small custard dishes on a rimmed baking sheet. In a small pan on medium heat, whisk together cream, sugar, and 2 tablespoons honey until simmering. Stir in seeds from vanilla bean. Stir in the vanilla pod. Stir in lemon peel. Let steep 5 minutes. Remove peel and vanilla pod. Stir in 5 tablespoons lemon juice. Divide custard evenly among dishes. Chill 1 hour.

2. In a bowl, whisk together remaining honey, lemon juice, and rum. Add berries (or mango). Stir to coat. Let sit 1 hour. Serve custard with fruit mixture on top.

Health Benefits of Honey

Acts as natural antibacterial and antifungal. Improves athletic performance when eaten before workouts. Soothes sore throats and relieves coughs.

70. Poached Pears with Pepper Ice Cream

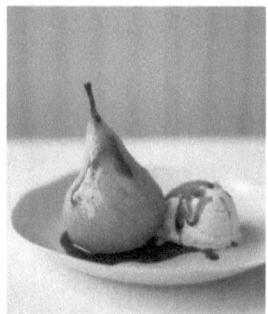

Try out this age-old recipe with a modern twist.

Ingredients

- 3 cups Whole Milk
- 1 cup (plus 1 Tbsp.) Heavy Cream
- 3 Tbsp. (plus 1 tsp.) Peppercorns
- 8 ½ large Egg Yolks
- 1 ¼ cup (plus 2 Tbsps.) Sugar
- 4 cups Pomegranate Juice
- 3-5 Dashes Black Pepper
- 8 Seckel Pears (peeled)
- 1 1/3 cup Almond Flour
- 2 large Eggs
- 8 ¾ Tbsp. Butter
- 1 Tbsp. Flour
- 4 oz. Cabrales Cheese (in 8 equal slices)

Method

1. In a medium pan on medium-high heat, whisk together cream, milk, and peppercorns. Cook until gently boiling. Remove from heat. Let sit 20 minutes. Strain mixture to remove peppercorns. Return to heat until gently boiling again. Remove from heat. Set aside.

2. In a bowl, whisk together egg yolks and ¾ cup sugar until pale. Whisk in ½ cup of milk mixture. Pour this egg mixture into the milk mixture. Cook over medium heat, stirring constantly with a wooden spoon. Do not let it boil. Remove from heat. Pour through a fine mesh sieve into a bowl. Set bowl in an ice bath. Stir frequently until completely cooled. Cover and refrigerate 4 hours. Process in an ice cream maker according to instructions. Freeze.

3. In a medium pan on medium-high heat, blend together pomegranate juice and black pepper until boiling. Add in the pears. Reduce heat to medium-low. Cook 15 minutes. Remove from heat. Let cool. Set pears aside in refrigerator. Return pomegranate mixture to a boil over medium-high heat. Cook 15 minutes. Pour through a fine sieve into a bowl. Let cool. Preheat oven to 375°F.

4. In a bowl, whisk together butter and ½ cup sugar until creamy. Add almond flour. Blend well. Whisk in eggs one at a time. Add 1 tablespoon flour. Whisk. Spread almond mixture into a greased baking dish. Bake 18-20 minutes. Let cool. Use a pastry cutter or knife to cut out 8 diamond shape pieces of the almond creams. Cut each poached pear in half crosswise. Remove core from bottom.

5. Stand each pear bottom on an individual serving plate. Top with a slice of cheese. Put pear tops on. Drizzle pomegranate sauce over them. Place an almond cream beside each pear. Top with a scoop of the prepared pepper ice cream.

Health Benefits of Pears

Improve heart health. Rich in antioxidants. High in fiber.

71. Hot Cocoa with Peppermint Ice Cream

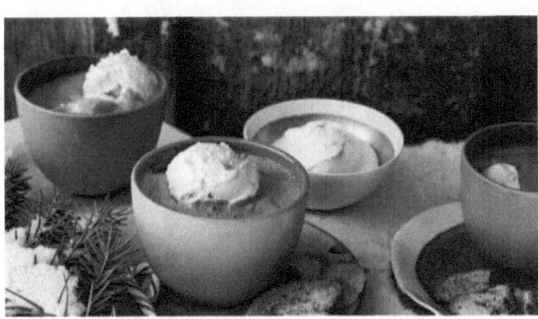

Hot cocoa and peppermint ice cream bringing out the best in each other in this recipe.

Ingredients

- 3 cups Whole Milk
- 1 cup Chilled Heavy Cream
- 1/3 cup Sugar

- 1/3 cup Unsweetened Cocoa Powder
- 2 pints Peppermint Ice Cream
- 5 oz. Dark Chocolate Chunks
- 1 Tbsp. Espresso or Dark Roast Coffee Grounds
- 1 Vanilla Bean (split lengthwise)
- 1 pinch Salt

Method

1. In a large pot, combine ½ cup cream, milk, ¼ cup water, sugar, and salt. Bring to a boil. Stir until sugar dissolves. Scrape out seeds from vanilla bean into milk. Add vanilla pod. Stir in chocolate chunks and cocoa powder. Whisk until melted and gently boiling.

2. In a bowl, whisk together remaining cream and coffee grounds to firm peaks. Remove vanilla pod and seeds from cocoa mixture. Discard. Pour mixture into a blender. Blend 2 minutes. Scoop ice cream into mugs. Divide cocoa evenly among the mugs. Top each with a dollop of whipped coffee cream.

Tips

Lower the sugar by replacing sugar with stevia or other natural sugar substitutes. Use almond milk in place of regular milk as a naturally sweet and healthier alternative. Use a teaspoon of vanilla extract if you don't have vanilla beans.

72. Buttermilk Panna Cotta with Apricot and Candied Fennel

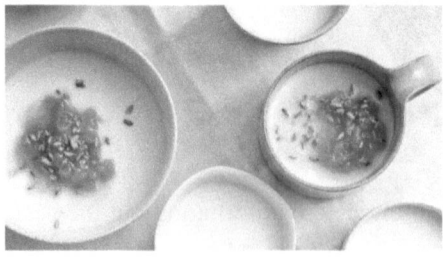

This unique dessert is simple yet elegant.

Ingredients

- 3 cups Buttermilk
- 2 ¾ cups Heavy Cream

- ¾ cup Dried Apricots (chopped)
- 2/3 cup Sugar
- 1 Tbsp. Fennel Seeds
- 2 ½ tsp Unflavored Gelatin Powder

Method

1. Sprinkle gelatin powder over a ¼ cup cold water. Let sit 10 minutes. In a pot over medium heat, heat ½ cup cream to 100°F. Remove from heat. Stir in gelatin and sugar. Whisk until dissolved. Gradually whisk in remaining cream and buttermilk. Divide mixture into 8 small custard dishes. Chill 4 hours.

2. In a small pot on high heat, boil 1 cup water, 2 tablespoons sugar, and apricots. Reduce heat. Simmer 20-25 minutes, stirring occasionally. In another pot, boil 2 tablespoons water with 1 tablespoon sugar on medium-high heat. Cook 4 minutes, stirring often.

3. Add fennels seeds. Reduce heat to medium. Cook 2 minutes, stirring constantly. Remove from heat, stir constantly 1-2 minutes. Transfer seeds to a bowl. Set aside. Top each panna cotta dish with apricot compote and sprinkle with fennel seeds.

Health Benefits of Apricot

Prevent age-related macular degeneration in the eyes. Lowers blood pressure. Helps speed up weight loss.

73. Frozen Ginger Vanilla Yogurt with Peach Compote

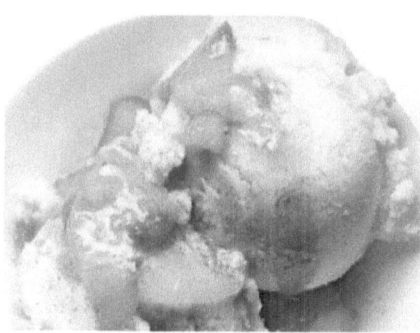

The hint of ginger really complements all the other flavors in this recipe.

Ingredients

- 2 cups Plain Greek Yogurt
- 3 cups Vanilla Pudding
- 2 large Peaches (pitted, sliced)
- 4 Tbsp. Honey
- 3 Tbsp. Sugar
- 1 tsp Vanilla Extract
- 2 tsp Fresh Ginger (grated)
- ½ tsp Cinnamon

Method

1. In a bowl, whisk together pudding, yogurt, honey, vanilla extract, and 1 teaspoon ginger until smooth. Freeze 4-6 hours. Remove from freezer. Let sit 15 minutes.

2. In a medium pan, boil 1 tablespoon water, remaining ginger, cinnamon, and peaches. Reduce heat. Simmer 4-5 minutes. Let cool. Pour yogurt mixture into a blender and pulse until smooth. Divide yogurt mixture into bowls. Top with peach mixture and sprinkle with cinnamon.

Health Benefits of Peaches

Help reduce anxiety. Help improve kidney and bladder health. Helps boost metabolism.

74. Cinnamon Bundt Cake

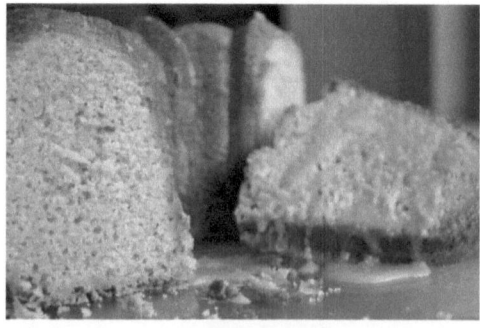

Cinnamon buns get a Bundt cake makeover in this recipe.

Ingredients

- 3 ½ cups Whole Grain Flour
- 2 ½ tsp Active Dry Yeast
- ¼ cup Warm Water
- ¼ cup Sugar
- 4 large Egg Yolks
- 10 Tbsps. Butter
- 1 1/8 tsp Salt
- 2/3 cup Brown Sugar
- 1 Tbsp. Cinnamon

Method

1. Dissolve yeast and 1 teaspoon sugar in warm water. Let sit 5 minutes. In another bowl, beat together sugar and butter until smooth. Beat in buttermilk, egg yolks, and salt until thoroughly combined. Beat in yeast mixture. Add flour 1 cup at a time until it forms a dough. Knead dough on a floured surface until smooth. Place dough in an oiled bowl. Cover with oiled plastic wrap. Let rise at room temperature until doubled in size.

2. In a bowl, combine brown sugar, cinnamon, and salt. Roll out dough into a (12"x18") rectangle. Brush the top with melted butter until well coated. Sprinkle sugar mixture evenly over the dough. Pick up one short end and gently roll the dough into a cylinder. Cut the cylinder into 10 pieces. Grease a Bundt dish and sprinkle with brown sugar. Arrange the cinnamon roll pieces (seam side down) in the dish. Cover with plastic wrap. Let rise 45 minutes. Remove plastic. Bake 35 minutes at 350°F.

Health Benefits of Cinnamon

Boosts metabolism. Helps improve body's ability to breakdown and use blood sugar. Improves cognitive function.

75. Peach Rosé Gelée

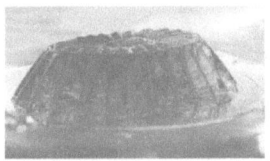

Upgrade Jell-O into a swanky dessert with this recipe.

Ingredients

- 3 cups Water
- 2 cups Sugar
- 4 ½ cups Rosé Wine
- 1 ¾ oz. Unflavored Gelatin Powder
- 2 Tbsps. Peach Schnapps

Method

1. In a small pot, combine 2 cups water with sugar. Sprinkle in gelatin. Let stand 1 minute. Cook on medium heat until dissolved, stirring occasionally. Remove from heat. Stir in schnapps, wine, and remaining water. Pour mixture into a mold. Cover. Chill 10 hours.

Tips

Use peach nectar instead of schnapps for a lower alcohol content. Use white grape juice instead of wine for a no alcohol version. Chop up 1-2 peaches and add it in for more texture and flavor.

76. Spiced Squash Pie with Pumpkin Seed Crumble

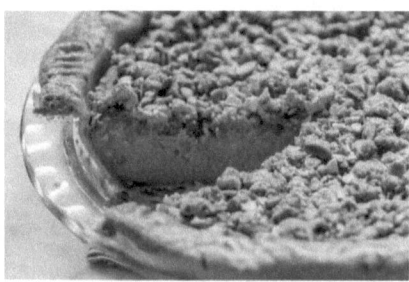

This dish revolutionizes the classic pumpkin pie.

Ingredients

- 1 ¼ cup Whole Grain Flour
- ¼ cup Cold Butter
- 2 tsp Sugar
- ½ tsp Salt
- 2 ½ lbs. Butternut Squash

- 1 ¼ cup Heavy Cream
- ½ cup Brown Sugar
- 2 Tbsps. Molasses
- 3 large Egg Yolks
- 1 large Egg
- 1 tsp Vanilla Extract
- ¾ tsp Ground Ginger
- ¾ tsp Cinnamon
- ½ tsp Salt
- ¼ tsp Nutmeg
- ½ cup Whole Grain Flour
- ½ cup Shelled Toasted Pumpkin Seeds (chopped)
- 1/3 cup Brown Sugar
- 6 Tbsps. Butter
- 1/8 tsp Baking Powder
- 1/8 tsp Salt
- ¼ tsp Cinnamon

Method

1. Preheat oven to 400°F. Place a rimmed baking sheet inside to preheat. In a food processor, pulse together flour, sugar, and salt. Add butter. Pulse until crumbly. Add 2 tablespoons cold water. Pulse until combined.

2. Gently knead dough on a floured surface. Flatten it into a disc Cover with plastic wrap. Chill 1 hour. Halve the squash. Remove seeds. Roast on preheated baking sheet 1 hour (cut side down). Let cool. Reduce oven to 375°F.

3. Roll out dough into a 13" circle. Press it into a 9" pie dish. Leave about 1" dough hanging over the edge. Trim away the rest. Chill 30 minutes.

4. In a bowl, whisk together ½ cup flour, 1/3 cup brown sugar, baking powder, salt, and cinnamon until combined. Add in 6 tablespoons butter. Massage together with hands until clumpy. Mix in pumpkin seeds. Chill 30 minutes.

5. Scoop out 2 ¼ cups squash flesh. Pulse in blender until smooth. Add molasses, ½ cup brown sugar, egg yolks, egg, ginger, nutmeg, cinnamon, vanilla, and salt. Pulse until creamy.

6. Pour squash puree into pie shell. Sprinkle over with pumpkin seed mixture. Place on preheated baking sheet. Cover crust edge in foil to prevent burning. Bake 1 hour (or until filling is set and topping is golden.

Health Benefits of Pumpkin Seeds

Rich in muscle-building magnesium. Rich in immune-boosting zinc. High in protein, fiber, and unsaturated fats making them the perfect weight loss tool.

77. Purple Rice Pudding with Rose Water Dates

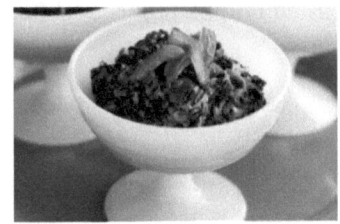

This dessert is remarkable for both its delicious flavor combinations and its striking appearance.

Ingredients

- ½ cup Black Rice
- 1 ¼ cup Water
- ¼ cup Pitted Dates (chopped)
- 2 Pitted Dates (sliced)
- 3 tsp Rose Water
- 1 ¼ cup Half and Half
- 2 Tbsps. Sugar
- 1 tsp Lemon Zest
- 1 Cinnamon Stick
- ½ tsp Vanilla Extract
- 1 pinch Salt

Method

1. Bring rice and water to a boil. Reduce heat. Simmer 30 minutes. In a bowl, toss together chopped dates with 2 teaspoons rose water. In another bowl, toss together sliced dates with remaining rose water. Set aside, stirring both bowls occasionally.

2. Add half & half, vanilla, ½ teaspoon zest, sugar, salt, and cinnamon stick to the rice. Mix well. Bring mixture to a boil over medium-high heat, stirring often. Reduce heat. Simmer 15 minutes, stirring occasionally. Remove from heat. Remove cinnamon stick. Stir in remaining zest and chopped dates. Divide into bowls. Garnish with date strips.

Health Benefits of Black Rice

Contains the same key antioxidants as blueberries. High in skin-nourishing vitamin E. High in fiber and key minerals.

78. Ginger Cream

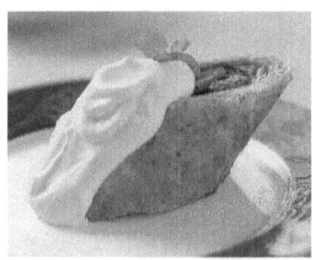

Use this zesty topping instead of plain whipped cream on pies, strudels, and anything else that calls for whipped cream.

Ingredients

- 1 cup Chilled Whipping Cream
- ¼ cup Water
- 1 ½ Tbsps. Sugar
- 3 Tbsps. Fresh Ginger (peeled, minced)

Method

1. In a small pot on medium heat, whisk together water, sugar, and ginger until dissolved. Simmer 5 minutes. Let cool. In a bowl, whip cream to soft peaks. Whisk in ginger mixture.

Health Benefits of Ginger

Helps your body absorb and use nutrients. Helps clear up sinuses and regulate mucus production. Helps treat nausea and upset stomach.

79. Italian Ice Cream Sandwiches

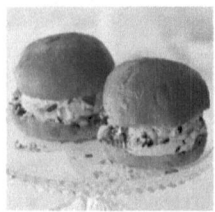

Try this literal interpretation of ice cream sandwiches on the next hot day.

Ingredients

- 2 Brioche Rolls
- 1 Pint Hazelnut Gelato
- 2 Tbsps. Dark Chocolate Chunks

Method

1. Slice brioche rolls, leaving them slightly attached. Tear out some of the bread from the middle to create small pockets for the gelato. Toast or grill rolls lightly (just until warm). Place a large scoop gelato into each roll. Sprinkle chocolate chunks over. Place roll top on. Serve.

Tips

Sprinkle in crushed hazelnuts for added flavor and texture. Drizzle a little honey on brioche rolls before toasting for more sweetness. Experiment with different ice cream flavors.

80. Mint Watermelon Ice Cubes

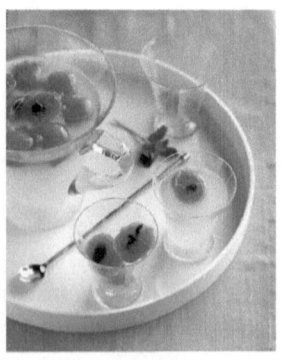

Use this recipe instead of boring water for your ice cubes and give every beverage a refreshing kick in the pants.

Ingredients

- 6 cups Watermelon (seeded, cubed)
- Sugar to taste
- Fresh Mint Leaves

Method

1. Puree watermelon in a blender. Mix in sugar to taste. Pour into ice cube trays. Top each cube with 1 mint leaf. Freeze.

Health Benefits of Watermelon

Eating the rinds helps burn fat and inhibit the storing of new fat. Improves kidney health. High potassium.

81. Chocolate Oatmeal Pie

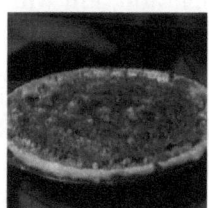

This unique pie recipe is as satisfying as it is nutritious.

Ingredients

- 1 ¼ cup Whole Grain Flour
- Egg White Glaze (1 Egg White Whisked with 1 tsp Water)
- ¼ lbs. Cold Butter (chopped)
- ½ cup Cold Water
- ½ cup Ice
- 2 Tbsps. Cider Vinegar
- 1 ½ tsp Sugar
- ½ tsp Salt
- 1 ½ cups Rolled Oats
- ¼ cup Heavy Cream
- 4 oz. Dark Chocolate (chopped)

- 4 large Eggs
- 1 cup Brown Sugar
- 2 Tbsps. Molasses
- 5 Tbsps. Butter
- 2 tsp Cider Vinegar
- 1 tsp Vanilla Extract
- ½ tsp Salt
- ¼ tsp Ground Ginger

Method

1. In a large bowl, combine flour, salt, and sugar. Add butter. Stir until crumbly. In another bowl, combine water, ice, and vinegar. Sprinkle 2 tablespoons over the flour mixture. Mix to combine. Add more water mixture 1 tablespoon at a time until dough comes together (but is still a little dry). Shape dough into a flat disc. Cover in plastic. Chill 1 hour.

2. Roll out dough into 13" circle. Press into 9" pie pan. Leave 1" overhang. Trim the rest. Chill 30 minutes. Preheat oven to 425°F. Line crust with aluminum foil. Fill with dry rice or pie weights. Bake 20 minutes.

3. Remove foil and weights. Let cool 3 minutes. Brush egg white glaze over crust. Bake 3 minutes. Let cool. Reduce heat to 350°F. Spread oats on a rimmed baking sheet. Toast 10 minutes, stirring occasionally. Let cool. Reduce temperature to 325°F.

4. In a pot over medium heat, bring cream to a boil. Remove from heat. Stir in chocolate. Let sit 5 minutes. Gently whisk until smooth. Pour chocolate mixture into pie shell. Place in freezer.

5. In a bowl, whisk together melted butter, ginger, brown sugar, and salt. Whisk in molasses, vanilla, and vinegar. Whisk in eggs one at a time. Stir in oats. Pour mixture into pie shell (once chocolate layer is set). Bake 1 hour (until filling is set and crust is golden and slightly puffy).

Health Benefits of Oatmeal

High in protein and fiber which curbs cravings and helps with weight loss. Lowers bad cholesterol. Eating oatmeal daily decreases risk of heart failure by up to 30%.

82. Curry Ginger Sugar Cookies

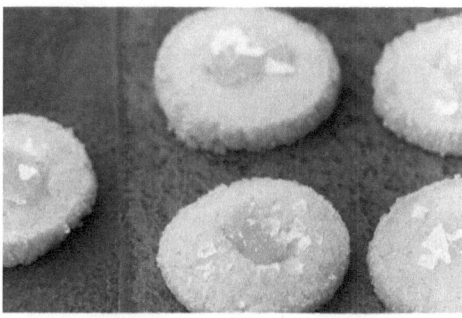

Liven up a stale sugar cookie recipe with a hint of curry and ginger.

Ingredients

- 24 1" slices Crystallized Ginger (halved)
- 1 ½ cups Whole Grain Flour
- ¾ cup Powdered Sugar
- 10 Tbsps. Cold Butter
- 1 large Egg
- 2 large Egg Yolks (beaten)
- Seeds from 1 Vanilla Bean
- 1 ½ tsp Ground Ginger
- 1 tsp Mild Curry Powder
- ½ tsp Salt
- Raw Sugar (for rolling)

Method

1. In a bowl, beat butter until thick and smooth. Whisk in vanilla seeds and egg. In a separate bowl, combine flour, powdered sugar, curry powder, ginger, and salt. Slowly add the dry ingredients to the wet ingredients until combined. Divide dough in half. Place each piece on separate parchment paper. Fold the paper over the dough and roll each into a (1 ½") log. Keep wrapped in paper. Chill until firm.

2. Preheat oven to 350°F. Line 2 baking sheets with parchment paper. Unwrap dough logs and brush beaten egg yolk over the surface. Roll logs in raw sugar. Cut into ¼" slices. Arrange slices on baking sheets. Press a piece of crystallized ginger into the center of each cookie. Bake 15 minutes.

Health Benefits of Curry Powder (Turmeric)

Acts as a powerful anti-inflammatory. Lowers blood pressure. Helps prevent food poisoning.

83. Cherry Almond Chocolate Bark

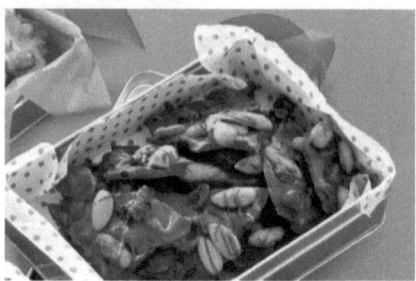

You won't be able to stop eating this delicious chocolate bark with cherry and almonds.

Ingredients

- 12 oz. Dark Chocolate
- ¾ cup Whole Almonds
- 1/3 cup Dried Tart Cherries (chopped)
- ½ tsp Vanilla Extract
- Toasted Almonds

Method

1. Preheat oven to 350°F. Spread almonds on a baking sheet lined with parchment paper. Toast 8-10 minutes. Let cool. Fill a medium pot on medium-low heat with 1" of water until simmering. Place a heatproof bowl on top of pot (without letting bottom of bowl touch water.

2. Place 10oz. of chocolate in the bowl. Stir until smooth. Remove bowl from pot. Add remaining chocolate to bowl. Stir in vanilla extract, cherries, and toasted almonds. Stir until coated. Spread mixture onto baking sheet. Chill 1 hour (until hardened). Break apart into pieces.

Health Benefits of Cherries

Provides natural pain relief. Helps treat migraines. Improves sleep quality.

84. Salted Caramel Risotto

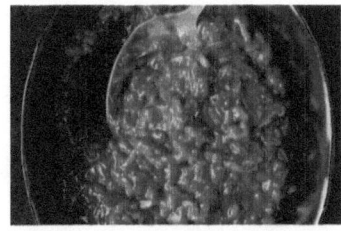

This simple dessert is a hearty and fulfilling final course.

Ingredients

- ½ cup Short Grain Rice
- 1 cup Whole Milk
- 1 cup Sugar
- 1 cup Cream
- ½ Tbsp. Butter
- 1 ½ tsp Vanilla Extract
- ½ tsp Salt
- Unsweetened Whipped Cream (for serving)

Method

1. Heat 2 cups of water over medium heat. In a large pot on medium-high heat, melt butter. When foamy, add rice. Cook 3-4 minutes, stirring constantly. Stir in heated water and milk. Bring to a boil. Reduce heat. Simmer 15 minutes, stirring occasionally.

2. In another large pot on high heat, mix together ¼ cup water with sugar. Stir until dissolved and boiling. Stop stirring. When golden streaks appear, swirl to blend until sugar caramelizes evenly. When caramelized sugar has been smoking for 15 seconds, remove from heat. Gradually whisk in cream until smooth. Stir the rice into the caramel cream. Simmer over medium-low heat 15-20 minutes, stirring often. Stir in vanilla and salt. Transfer to a bowl. Chill 30 minutes.

Tips

Serve this hot on top of vanilla ice cream. Stir in ½ cup crumbled almonds after cooking for more crunch. Add a dash or two of cinnamon to kick things up a notch.

85. Chocolate Dipped Candied Orange Peels

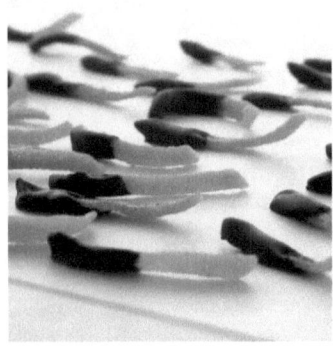

Enjoy all the health benefits of orange peels with the rich flavor of chocolate.

Ingredients

- 5 oranges
- 2 1/3 cups Sugar
- Water
- Salt
- 10.5 oz. Dark Chocolate

Method

1. Wash oranges. Use a peeler to peel away orange peel. Bring 4 cups water, orange peels, and a dash of salt to a boil. Boil 5 minutes. Drain. Repeat 1 more time.

2. In another pot, bring 1 2/3 cups water and 1 cup sugar to a boil. Stir until dissolved. Stir in orange peels. Remove from heat. Cover and let rest overnight. Remove the peels. Add 1/3 cup sugar to the syrup. Bring to a boil. Put orange peels back in. Remove from heat. Let rest overnight. Repeat this 3 more times. Let candied peels drain slowly at room temperature for 1 day. Cut into thin pieces.

3. Fill a medium pot with 1" water. Simmer on medium heat. Place a large bowl on top (don't let bottom touch water). Add chocolate. Stir until smooth. Use a fork to dip candied orange peel pieces into chocolate. Arrange dipped pieces on a plate or baking sheet. Chill 10 minutes.

Health Benefits of Orange Peel

Helps with respiratory problems. Chewing orange peels naturally whitens teeth and kills bad breath. Helps speed up weight loss.

86. Strawberry Black Pepper Truffles

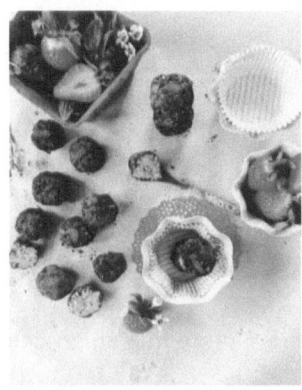

These simple little truffles are easy to make and uniquely delicious.

Ingredients

- 2/3 cup Heavy Cream
- 12 oz. Milk Chocolate (chopped)
- 1 ½ cups Freeze-Dried Strawberries
- 1 Tbsp. Black Pepper

Method

1. Heat a medium pot with 1-2" water over medium heat. Simmer. Place a large bowl on top (don't let bowl touch water). Add cream to bowl. Stir 3 minutes. Add chocolate. Stir until melted and combined. Remove bowl from heat. Let cool 15 minutes. Then freeze 1 hour. Use a melon baller or teaspoon to scoop out hardened truffle mixture onto a baking sheet lined with parchment paper.

2. Roll truffle balls in your hands quickly to form them into balls. This will get a little messy. Freeze truffle balls 20 minutes. Place strawberries in a Ziploc bag. Crush with a rolling pin until crumbly and partially pulverized. Pour into a bowl. Stir in pepper. Press and roll truffle balls in the strawberry mixture until coated.

Health Benefits of Black Pepper

Acts as a natural antibacterial. Helps treat digestive problems. Acts as a natural decongestant.

87. Strawberry S'mores

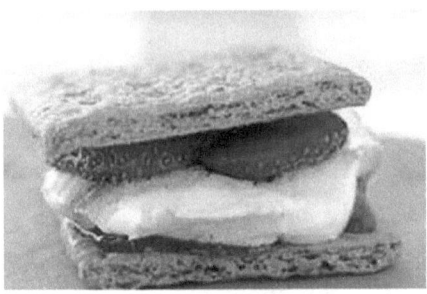

This recipe turns the campfire S'more into an upscale dessert.

Ingredients

- 12 medium Strawberries
- 8 large Marshmallows
- 8 slices Baguette
- 1 (4 oz.) bar Dark Chocolate (cut in 8 pieces)
- ¼ tsp Salt
- Olive Oil

Method

1. Prepare one side of your grill with a medium fire. Place strawberries and marshmallows on skewers (in alternating pattern). Lightly brush them with olive oil.

2. Place skewers over fire 4-5 minutes. Place baguette slices over the fire. Grill 1 minute. Move slices over to the other side of the grill (without the fire). Place a piece of chocolate on top of each slice. Sprinkle lightly with salt. Let chocolate soften slightly. Top each piece with a marshmallow and strawberry.

Health Benefits of Strawberries

Boost metabolism. Improve memory. High in heart-healthy potassium.

88. Honey Molasses Glazed Oranges

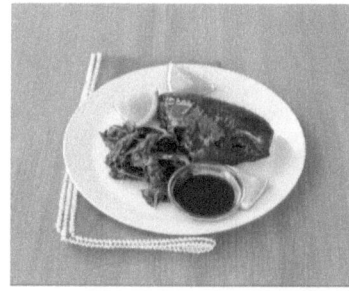

Honey and molasses combine for a rich glaze on these oranges.

Ingredients

- 8 large Navel Oranges (peeled, sliced into rounds)
- ¼ cup Honey
- 3 Tbsps. Molasses
- 8 large Dates (pitted, chopped)
- ½ tsp Cinnamon
- ¼ tsp Salt

Method

1. Arrange orange slices on a platter so that they are overlapping slightly. In a bowl, whisk together honey, molasses, cinnamon, and salt until well blended. Drizzle over orange slices. Sprinkle with dates.

Health Benefits of Molasses

High in iron. High in calcium. Works as a healthier alternative to refined sugar.

89. Walnut Amaranth Cookies

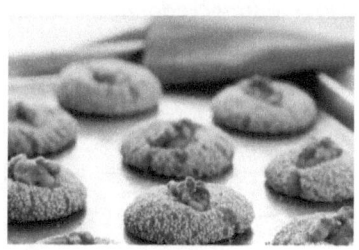

These scrumptious cookies are the healthiest solution to your nagging sweet tooth.

Ingredients

- ¾ cup Whole Grain Flour
- ¼ cup Amaranth Flour
- ½ cup Sugar
- 4 oz. Toasted Walnut Pieces
- 7 Tbsps. Butter
- 1 large Egg Yolk
- 1 Tbsp. Brandy
- 1 tsp Vanilla Extract
- ¼ tsp Salt
- 6 Tbsps. Amaranth Seeds (for rolling)
- 32 Toasted Walnut Halves (for topping)

Method

1. In a food processor, pulse together walnut pieces with 2 tablespoons sugar until ground into a powder. In a bowl, combine amaranth flour, salt, and flour. In another bowl, beat butter until smooth and fluffy. Whisk in brandy, egg yolk, and vanilla. Slowly whisk in ground walnuts. Slowly blend in amaranth flour mixture until combined. Cover and chill 3 hours. Preheat oven to 350°F.

2. Pinch off small (walnut-sized) pieces of dough. Roll into balls. Dip into amaranth seeds. Arrange on 2 parchment lined baking sheets. Press down on each ball to make an indentation in the center. Lightly press a walnut halve into the center. Bake each sheet of cookies separately for 17-18 minutes each.

Health Benefits of Amaranth

High in lysine which helps strengthen hair and prevent hair loss. Helps control appetite. High in bone-strengthening calcium.

90. Rose Prosecco Pops

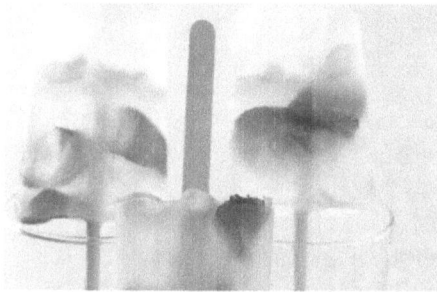

Popsicles aren't just for kids anymore. This recipe turns them into elegantly simple treats.

Ingredients

- 2 cups Cold, Flat Prosecco
- 1/3 cup Rose Water
- 1 ½ tsp Fresh Lemon Juice
- 30 or so Rosebud Petals (rinsed)
- Popsicle molds

Method

1. In a bowl, stir together prosecco, rose water, and lemon juice. Pour into Popsicle molds until 1/3 full. Drop 2-3 rose petals into each mold. Freeze 30 minutes. Remove. Fill molds another 1/3 of the way full. Add a couple rose petals. Insert sticks. Freeze. Remove. Fill the rest of the way. Add remaining rose petals. Freeze 8 hours.

Health Benefits of Rose Petals

High in Vitamin C. Helps digestion. Low in calories.

91. Greek Yogurt Topped with Cherries & Almond Syrup

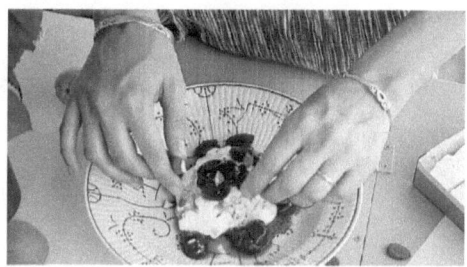

This rich dessert is nutritious and flavorful.

Ingredients

- 4 cups Red or Black Cherries (pitted)
- ¼ cup Almond Syrup
- ¼ cup Sugar
- 1 cup Whole Raw Almonds (chopped)
- 2 Tbsps. Fresh Lemon Juice
- 7 cups Plain Greek Yogurt

Method

1. In a pot on medium-high heat, mix ¼ cup water, sugar, lemon juice, almond syrup, and cherries. Stir until dissolved. Simmer 5 minutes. Let cool. When cooled, chill in fridge until completely cold. Divide yogurt into bowls. Top with cherry mixture. Garnish with almonds.

Tips

This dish is already super healthy. But you can make it even healthier by omitting the sugar. Use a blend of almonds and hazelnut for a richer flavor. Try vanilla Greek yogurt for added sweetness.

92. Berry Plum Pudding

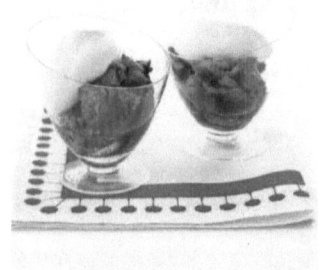

You'll enjoy the vibrant colors as much as you enjoy the bold flavors of this pudding.

Ingredients

- 12 oz. Red or Purple Plums (pitted, thinly sliced)
- 2 2/3 cups Raspberries

- 1 1/3 cups Blueberries
- 12 Egg Bread Slices (½" thick)
- ¾ cup Sugar
- 1 tsp Fresh Lemon Juice
- Ginger Cream

Method

1. Line 6 custard dishes with plastic wrap (leave about 3" of plastic wrap hanging over edges). Cut out circles from each bread slice (the same size as the bottom of the custard dishes.

2. In a medium pot over medium-low heat, mix plums and sugar. Stir until sugar dissolves. Simmer 5 minutes. Stir in the berries. Simmer 5 minutes. Stir in lemon juice. Remove from heat. Let cool. Place 2 plum slices at the bottom of each custard dish. Top with 2 tablespoons of fruit mixture. Press a bread circle on top.

3. Divide the rest of the fruit mixture evenly into the custard dishes. Cover with remaining bread circles. Press down firmly. Cover with the plastic. Arrange dishes on a baking sheet. Rest another baking sheet on top. Weigh down top with heavy cans or other weights. Chill overnight.

Health Benefits of Berries

Improve cognitive function. Help lower your risk for cancer. Help control appetite and speed weight loss.

93. Cranberry Pistachio Oatmeal Ice Box Cookies

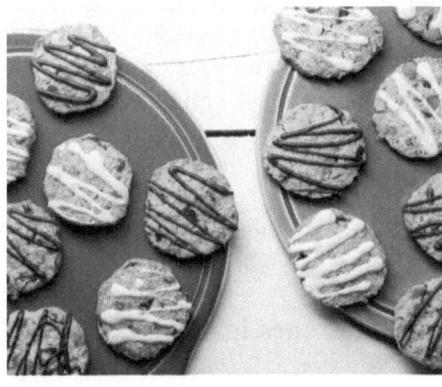

Always keep a batch of this healthy, scrumptious cookie dough on hand in your freezer for a quick dessert.

Ingredients

- 1 cup Butter (softened)
- 1 cup Brown Sugar
- 2/3 cup Sugar
- 1 cup Roasted Salted Pistachios
- 1 cup Dried Cranberries
- 3 cups Rolled Oats
- 1 ½ cups Whole Grain Flour
- 2 large Eggs
- 1 ½ tsp Vanilla Extract
- 1 tsp Baking Powder
- ½ tsp Cinnamon
- ¼ tsp Nutmeg
- ¼ tsp Salt

Method

1. In a bowl, beat together butter, sugar, and brown sugar until fluffy and light. Whisk in baking powder, baking soda, cinnamon, nutmeg, and salt. Whisk in eggs and vanilla.

2. Stir in flour until well combined. Stir in cranberries, pistachios, and oats until evenly distributed. Separate dough into 4 pieces. Place each on a separate piece of parchment paper. Fold paper over and roll the dough into 9" long cylinders.

3. Keep wrapped in paper. Wrap plastic wrap over that. Twist ends tightly to seal. Chill 4 hours (or store for later use). Remove cookie log, cut into ¼" slices. Arrange slices on baking sheets lined with parchment paper. Bake for 8-10 minutes at 350°F.

Health Benefits of Pistachios

Lower bad cholesterol. High in bone-strengthening phosphorus. Improves sleep quality.

94. Grilled Peaches in Herb & Lime Syrup

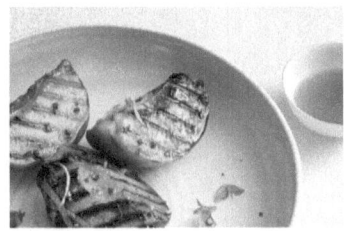

This dish kicks off with the bold flavor of the herb & lime syrup and then rounds off with the subtle sweetness of the grilled peaches.

Ingredients

- 4 large Peaches (pitted, quartered)
- ½ cup Brown Sugar
- ¼ cup Water
- ¼ cup Fresh Lime Juice
- ¼ cup Fresh Basil Leaves
- Black Pepper
- Coconut Oil (or Olive Oil)

Method

1. In a pot over medium heat, combine brown sugar and water. Stir until dissolved. Turn off heat. Stir in lime juice and basil. Let stand 15 minutes. Remove basil leaves.

2. Set a grill to medium heat. Sprinkle peach wedges with brown sugar. Grill each wedge (cut side down) 2 minutes each cut side. Transfer to serving bowls. Sprinkle with pepper and spoon basil syrup over. Garnish with fresh basil leaves.

Health Benefits of Basil

High in muscle-building magnesium. High in antioxidants. Acts as a natural antibacterial treatment.

Special BONUS Recipes!

Firstly, I'd like to congratulate you for grabbing a copy of this book! Here are some extra special bonus dessert recipes that I have added for you – they are extra special and great for any holiday season!

Important Note

A lot of the recipes require the use of "sugar-free powdered sugar". You can use sugar instead of this, but if you would like to keep the recipe really healthy, you can substitute it for the following – sugar-free powdered sugar. The recipe to make this is:

- 1 cup corn starch
- 1 cup powdered milk
- 1 cup Stevia

Simply grind these ingredients together in a blender and it will yield 1 ¾ cup of sugar-free powdered sugar. Now that that's out of the way, let's get into it! Enjoy the bonuses!

95. Peanut Butter Eggs

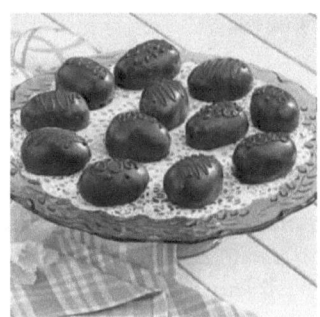

Ingredients (makes 8 medium sized eggs)

- ¼ cup peanut butter
- Dash sea salt
- ¼ cup sugar free powdered sugar
- 2 tbsp cocoa powder
- 2 tbsp virgin coconut oil
- 2 tbsp pure maple syrup

Method

1. Combine peanut butter, salt, and powdered sugar in a mixing bowl. Mix until you get a dough consistency. Form the dough into egg shapes and place on a tray. Chill eggs in the freezer for an hour or until dough is firm.

2. While the dough is chilling, combine in a bowl the cocoa powder, coconut oil, and maple syrup until a liquidy consistency is formed. After eggs have chilled, coat each egg in the chocolate liquid and return eggs back to freezer until chocolate is fully hardened.

96. Fruit Pizza Pie

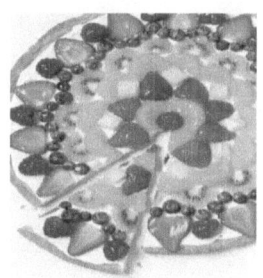

Ingredients

For the Pie Base (makes 1 medium size pizza pie)

- ½ cup white flour
- 1 tsp baking powder
- A pinch of stevia
- ½ cup low fat milk or substitute with almond milk
- 2 tbsp. applesauce
- A small pinch of sea salt
- ½ tsp vanilla extract
- A dash of cinnamon
- Choice of fruit and nuts (chopped almonds or walnuts, raisins, mandarin oranges, kiwi, mixed berries, and apples)

For the Optional Cream Cheese Frosting

- ¼ cup fat free cream cheese
- ½ tsp vanilla extract
- A dash of stevia
- 2 tsp milk

Method

1. Mix all ingredients, and pour into a greased pie plate or tin. Place in a 420F oven for ten minutes or less. After pie has cooled enjoy! To take your pie to the next level, you can add a healthy cream cheese frosting

and add more fresh fruit on top. Simply whip frosting ingredients with a beater.

97. Coconut Muffin Cake

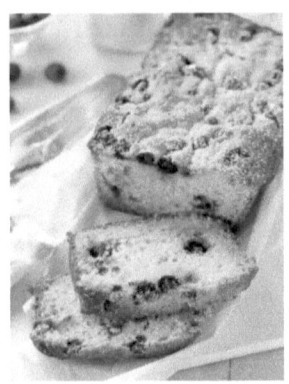

Ingredients (makes 12 muffins/1 loaf)

- 1 cup white flour
- ¼ tsp cinnamon
- 1 tsp baking powder
- A dash of sea salt
- ½ tsp baking soda
- 2 tsp ground flaxseed
- ¼ cup plus 2 tbsp xylitol
- ⅛ tsp stevia
- 2 tsp vanilla extract
- 1 cup crushed & drained pineapple
- ½ cup low fat canned coconut milk or substitute almond milk
- Shredded coconut
- ¼ cup chopped walnuts

Method

1. Preheat oven to 350F. In a bowl combine, flour, cinnamon, baking powder, sea salt, baking soda, flaxseed, chopped walnuts, xylitol, and stevia. Set aside.

2. In a separate bowl combine pineapple and coconut or almond milk. Slowly add the dry ingredients from step 1 to wet while stirring continuously to form batter. Pour batter into a greased cupcake tin or

loaf tin, and bake for 35 minutes. Allow to cool. Then sprinkle shredded coconut over muffins and enjoy!

98. Mini Carrot Cake

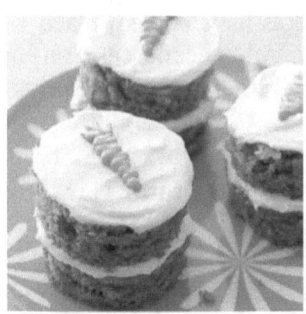

Ingredients for Cake (serves 2)

- ¼ cup white flour
- ⅛ tsp baking soda
- ½ tsp cinnamon
- A dash of sea salt
- ¼ tsp baking powder
- 2 tsp ground flaxseed
- 1 ½ tbsp xylitol
- A pinch of stevia
- 1 small fresh carrot (steamed and mashed)
- 1 tbsp fat free milk or almond milk
- 1 tbsp coconut oil
- ¼ tsp vanilla extract
- Chopped walnuts

For the Optional Cream Cheese Frosting

- ¼ cup fat free cream cheese
- ½ tsp vanilla extract
- A dash of stevia
- 2 tsp milk

Method

1. Preheat oven 350F. In a bowl combine flour, baking soda, cinnamon, sea salt, baking powder flaxseed xylitol, and stevia. Set aside. In a

separate bowl beat together mashed carrots, milk, oil, and vanilla extract. Then slowly add the dry ingredients from step 1.

2. Pour half and half into 2 greased soufflé dishes, and bake in oven for 15 minutes. Let cake cool, and beat frosting ingredients together in a bowl. After the cakes have cooled, place 1 cake on a tray and spread frosting on evenly. Add second cake on top of already frosted cake, and finish frosting. To add a garnish, sprinkle chopped walnuts on top of frosted cake.

99. Lemon Bars

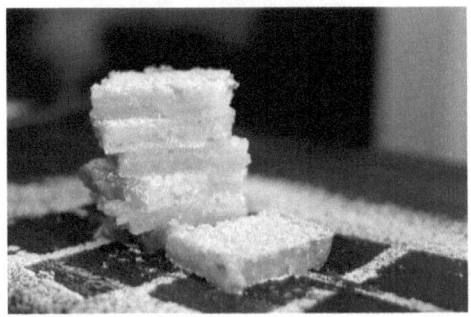

Ingredients

For the Crust

- 1 cup white flour
- ¼ cup sugar free powdered sugar (instructions in the introduction)
- A dash of sea salt
- ¼ cup coconut oil
- 1 ½ tbsp water

For the Filling

- ½ tbsp cornstarch
- ¼ cup lemon juice (add a little more if you prefer a stronger lemon flavor)
- ¼ cup sugar free powdered sugar
- 2 tbsp sugar free powdered sugar (instructions in the introduction)
- 1 cup lite tofu
- Zest of one lemon
- A few drops yellow food coloring

Method

1. Preheat oven to 350F. In a bowl, combine crust ingredients and mix by hand. Grease a 8x8 tin, and press crust evenly into the bottom. Bake crust in oven for 10 minutes. Beat filling ingredients, pour into crust, and bake for another 25 minutes. Allow to cool and serve.

100. Snickerdoodle Bars

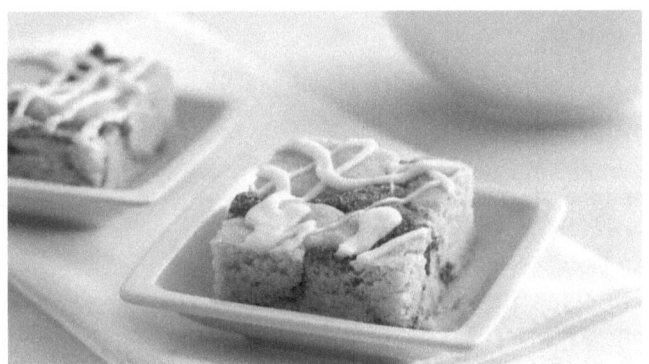

Ingredients

- 1 ½ cups chickpeas (boiled, rinsed, drained, and mashed)
- 3 tbsp. almond butter
- ¾ tsp baking powder
- 1-2 tsp vanilla extract
- ⅛ tsp baking soda
- Sea salt to taste
- ¾ cup xylitol
- 1 tbsp. applesauce
- ¼ cup ground flaxseed
- 2 tsp cinnamon
- Chopped walnuts
- Raisins

Method

1. Preheat oven to 350F. In a bowl, combine all ingredients and mix until dough forms. In a greased 8x8 pan, scoop dough and press into the bottom. Bake for 30 min and allow to cool.

101. Sugar Cookies

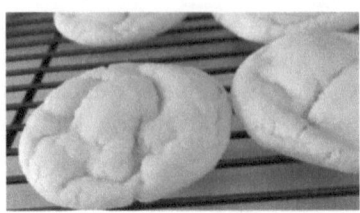

Ingredients

- ¾ cup white flour
- ¼ tsp baking powder
- ¼ tsp salt
- ¼ tsp baking soda
- ¼ cup xylitol
- ½ tsp vanilla extract
- 1 ½ tbsp. low fat milk or almond milk
- ¼ cup applesauce

Method

1. Preheat oven to 325F. In a bowl, combine flour, baking soda, salt, baking powder, and xylitol. In a separate bowl, combine vanilla milk, and applesauce. Slowly, while mixing, add the dry ingredients to the wet ingredients until a dough forms.

2. Roll the dough into balls, flatten with a fork, place on a tray, and chill for about 15 minutes. Then place cookies on a baking sheet, and bake for about 10 minutes (when the cookies are taken out of the oven they will look underdone, just allow to set for 5 minutes).

102. Breakfast Carrot Waffles

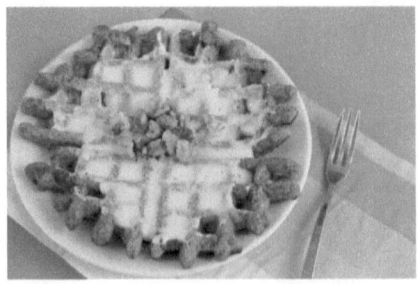

Ingredients (makes 2 waffles)

- ½ cup white flour
- ½ tsp cinnamon
- ¼ tsp salt
- ¼ tsp baking soda
- 1 tsp baking powder
- 2 tbsp. pure maple syrup
- ¼ cup shredded carrot
- ⅓ cup low fat milk or almond milk
- 1 tbsp. coconut oil
- 1 tsp vanilla extract

Method

1. Grease and preheat waffle iron. In a bowl, combine flour, cinnamon, salt, baking soda, and baking powder. Mix well. In a separate bowl combine carrot, milk, oil, syrup, and vanilla. Slowly, while stirring, add the dry ingredients to the wet. Continue stirring until a smooth batter is formed. Pour half the batter into the iron, wait till the waffle is finished cooking, serve, and enjoy!

103. Coffee Cream Cheese Cake

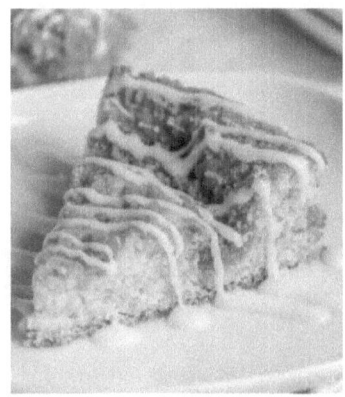

Ingredients

For the Cake

- ¾ cup low fat milk or almond milk
- 1 tbsp apple cider vinegar

- 2 cups white flour
- ½ tsp baking soda
- 2 tsp baking powder
- ½ tsp. salt
- ½ tsp. cinnamon
- ½ cup coconut oil
- 1 cup xylitol

For the Frosting

- 1 8-oz container low cream cheese
- ⅓ cup xylitol
- 2 tbsp. white flour
- 2 tsp lemon zest
- ½ tsp salt
- ½ tsp vanilla extract

For the Topping

- ⅔ cup coconut brown sugar
- ½ cup white flour
- 1 tsp cinnamon
- ¼ tsp nutmeg
- ½ tsp salt
- ⅔ cup applesauce

Method

1. Preheat oven to 350F, and grease a 8x8 tin. In a bowl, combine the vinegar, milk, and xylitol from the cake ingredients and set aside. In a separate bowl, combine the flour, baking soda, baking powder, salt, cinnamon, and oil from the cake ingredients. Slowly, while stirring, add the dry ingredients to the wet until a batter forms.

2. Pour half the batter into the greased tin. In a separate bowl combine the cream cheese, xylitol, flour, lemon zest, salt, and vanilla. Drop spoonfuls of the filling into spots in the batter, and then pour the rest of the batter into the tin. In a separate bowl, combine the topping ingredients and mix into a crumble. Sprinkle the crumble over the batter. Bake for 45 minutes.

104. Chocolate Tart

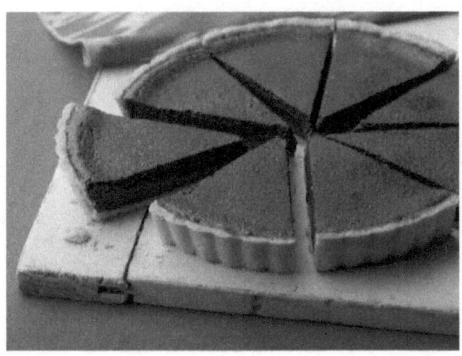

Ingredients

For the Crust

- 1 cup pitted dates
- 1 cup ground almonds
- 1 tsp vanilla extract
- 2 tbsp cocoa

For the Pudding

- 4 avocados
- A dash of sea salt
- 1 tbsp vanilla extract
- ¼ cup maple syrup
- ⅓ cup cocoa
- ½ cup melted dark chocolate chips

Method

1. Add pitted dates and almonds to a blender and grind. In a bowl add the ground dates and almonds, vanilla, and cocoa. Mix until a dough consistency is formed. Grease a muffin tin, and press the crust into the tin.

2. In a bowl, combine the avocado, sea salt, vanilla, syrup, cocoa, and melted chips from the pudding ingredients. Blend until a liquid consistency is reached. Pour pudding over crust, and chill in the freezer.

105. No Bake Key Lime Pie Bars

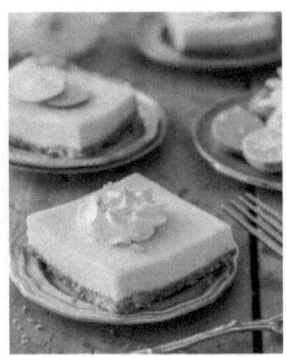

Ingredients

For the Crust

- 1 cup pitted dates
- 1 cup shredded coconut
- 1 cup chopped cashews
- 1 tsp vanilla extract

For the Filling

- 2 cups almond butter
- 1 tsp vanilla extract
- 2 tbsp. honey
- 6 tsp stevia
- Zest of 1/2 lime
- Juice of 1/2 lime
- Extra lime zest for topping

Method

1. In a blender combine the dates, coconut, cashews, and vanilla extract from the crust ingredients. Remove from blender, and press dough mixture into an 8x8-greased pan.

2. In a separate bowl, combine almond butter, vanilla, honey, stevia, juice from a lime, and zest from a lime. Mix together, pour over crust, sprinkle zest on top, and freeze overnight.

106. No Bake Gingerbread Cookies & Creamy Frosting

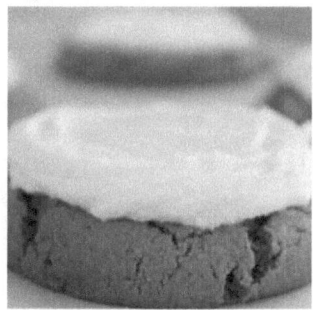

Ingredients

For the Gingerbread Balls

- 2 cups ground cashews
- ½ cup ground flaxseed
- ½ cup almond flour
- ½ tbsp ginger powder
- 1 tsp pumpkin pie spice
- 1 tbsp. vanilla
- 1 cup pitted dates (soaked & drained)
- ¼ cup molasses

For the Frosting

- ¼ cup fat free cream cheese
- ½ tsp vanilla extract
- A dash of stevia
- 2 tsp milk

Method

1. In a bowl, combine cashews, flaxseed, flour, ginger powder, and pumpkin pie spice. Mix well. In a separate bowl, combine vanilla dates and molasses. Mix well. Slowly, while stirring, pour the dry ingredients into the wet and mix until a dough consistency is formed.

2. Form medium size balls using the dough, and place on a tray. Using a fork flatten the balls, and place in the refrigerator for 2 hours. In a separate bowl, combine the frosting ingredients and whip till fluffy. Add a dollop of frosting to the top of each ball.

107. Pumpkin Pie Cheesecakes

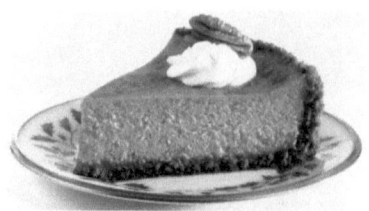

Ingredients

For the Crust

- 1 cup shredded coconut
- 1 ¼ cup chopped pecans
- 1 cup pitted dates (soaked and drained)
- 1 tsp vanilla extract

For the Filling

- ¾ cup pumpkin puree
- ½ cup almond butter
- 1 tsp vanilla extract
- 1 tsp cinnamon
- ¼ tsp ginger powder
- ⅛ tsp cloves
- 3 tbsp maple syrup
- 2 tbsp stevia
- pinch of sea salt

Method

1. In a large bowl, combine crust ingredients and mix until a dough consistency is formed. In a greased 8x8 pan, press dough evenly into the bottom. In a separate bowl combine cinnamon, ginger powder, cloves, stevia, and salt. Mix well.

2. In a separate bowl, combine pumpkin puree, almond butter, vanilla, and syrup. Mix well. Slowly, while stirring, add the dry ingredients to the wet and stir. Pour filling onto the crust, top with extra pecans if you like, and freeze overnight.

108. Apple Crumble Cupcakes

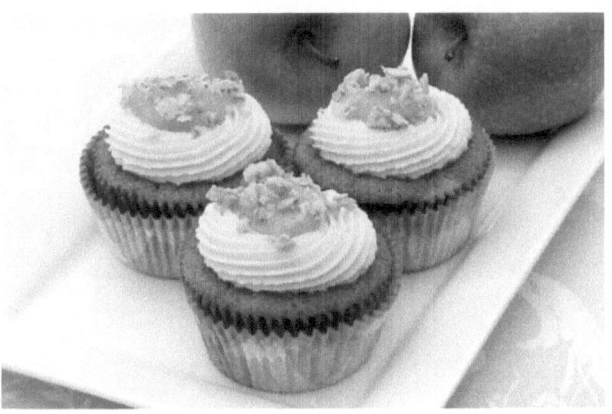

Ingredients (12 muffins)

- 1 cup almond flour
- 12 tsp stevia
- 1 tsp cinnamon
- 1 tsp nutmeg
- ½ tsp baking soda
- ¼ tsp sea salt
- 4 egg whites
- ½ cup water
- 3 apples (peeled and chopped finely)
- ⅓ cup plain non-fat Greek yogurt
- 1 tbsp vanilla extract

Method

1. Preheat oven to 350F. In a bowl, combine flour, stevia, cinnamon, nutmeg, baking soda, and salt. Mix well. In a separate bowl combine egg whites, water, apples, yogurt, and vanilla. Mix well. Slowly, while mixing, add the dry ingredients to wet and mix well until a batter consistency is formed. Pour batter into a greased muffin tin, and bake for 25 minutes. Allow to cool before serving.

109. Traditional Strawberry Short Cake

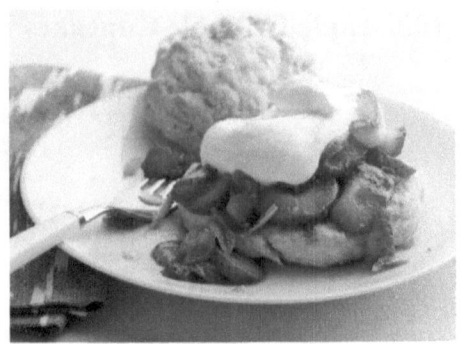

Ingredients

- 1 tbsp. stevia
- 1 tbsp. cornstarch
- 1 cup orange juice
- ¼ tsp vanilla extract
- 1 ½ cups sliced fresh strawberries
- 6 sponge cake dessert shells

Method

1. In a saucepan on medium heat, combine stevia and cornstarch. Stir in orange juice, bring mixture to a boil, and continue until mixture has thickened (1 minute after boiling. Remove from heat. Let mixture cool completely. Add vanilla and strawberries into the mixture. Mix well and spoon over the desert shells.

110. Fudge Brownies & Cream Cheese Frosting

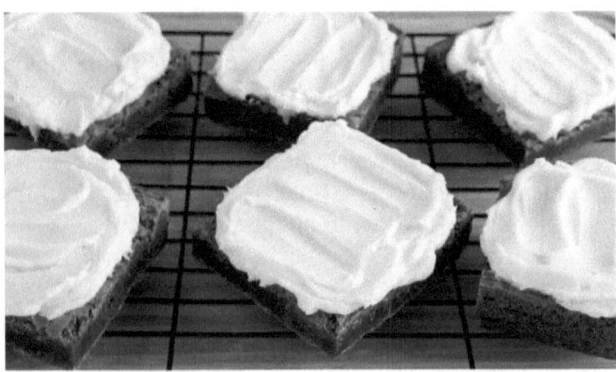

Ingredients

For the Brownie Batter

- ¾ cup stevia
- ¼ cup low fat butter
- 1 large egg
- 1 large egg white
- 1 tbsp. vanilla extract
- ½ cup almond flour
- ¼ cup cocoa

For the Cream Cheese Frosting

- 1 container fat free cream cheese
- ¼ cup stevia
- 3 tbsp. fat free milk or almond milk

Method

1. Preheat oven to 350F. In a bowl, combine butter, egg, egg white, vanilla, and stevia. Mix Well. Slowly, while stirring, add the cocoa and almond flour until a batter consistency is formed. Pour batter into a greased 8x8 tin.

2. In a separate bowl, beat together cream cheese, stevia, and almond milk until smooth consistency is formed. Pour frosting over brownie batter, and using a toothpick create a marble effect by swirling the brown batter into the frosting. Bake for 35 min.

111. Chilled Peanut Butter Pie

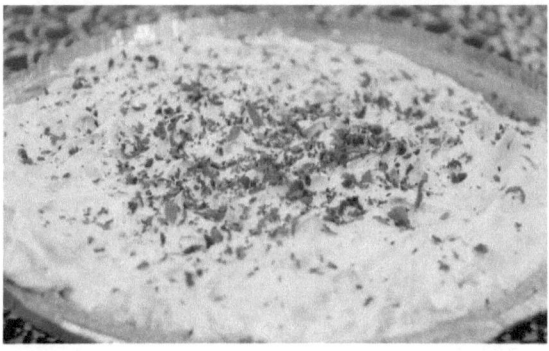

Ingredients

For the Crust

- 1 ⅔ cups chocolate graham cracker crumbs
- 3 tbsp. stevia
- 2 large egg whites

For the Filling

- 4 tbsp. stevia
- 1 ¼ fat free milk or almond milk
- ⅔ cup crunchy peanut butter
- ½ tsp vanilla
- ½ cup fat-free cream cheese
- 1 container frozen fat-free whipped topping (thawed)
- 3 tbsp. finely chopped peanuts

Method

1. Preheat oven to 350F. In a bowl, combine egg whites, graham cracker crumbs, and stevia. Mix. Press into the bottom of a greased pie plate, and bake for 10 minutes. In a saucepan over medium heat, combine milk sugar and cook for 2 minutes while continuously stirring. In a bowl, add heated mixture, peanut butter, and vanilla. Whisk together and chill in the refrigerator for 30 minutes.

2. In a bowl add cream cheese and chilled mixture and beat until fluffy. Mix in the whipped topping, pour into pie plate, sprinkle chopped peanuts on top, and chill overnight.

112. Vanilla Angel Food Cake

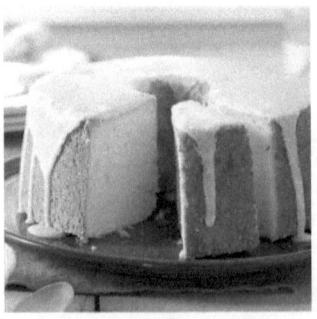

Ingredients

- 1 ½ cups stevia
- 1 tsp vanilla extract
- 1 cup sifted cake flour
- 12 large egg whites
- ½ tsp cream of tartar
- ¼ tsp salt
- 1 tsp lemon juice

Method

1. Preheat oven to 325F. In a bowl, combine flour, half of the stevia, and egg whites. Beat mixture, add cream of tartar, salt, and lemon juice, and continue beating while slowly adding the rest of the stevia.

2. Pour flour mixture over egg white mixture a little bit at a time. Pour the batter into an ungreased tube pan. Bake for 50 minutes or until cake springs back when lightly touched. Tip pan upside down on a tray, and allow to cool. Pull angel food cake out of the tin by shaking side to side when cooled and serve.

113. Chocolate Truffles

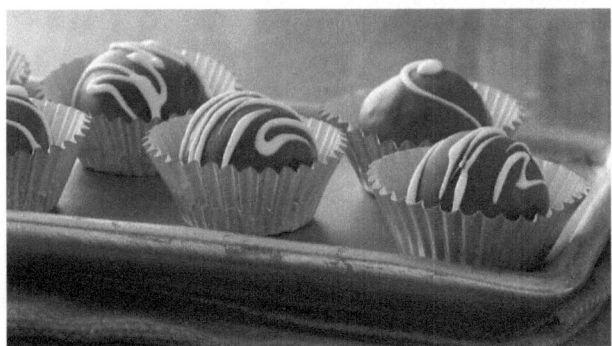

Ingredients

- 1 cup coconut oil
- ½ cup Cocoa powder
- ¼ maple syrup
- 2 tsp hazelnut extract
- ½ tsp vanilla extract

Method

1. In a bowl, combine all ingredients and beat together. Using a spoon, scoop medium size balls into a muffin tray and chill in the fridge overnight.

114. Chilled Creamy Orange Tarts

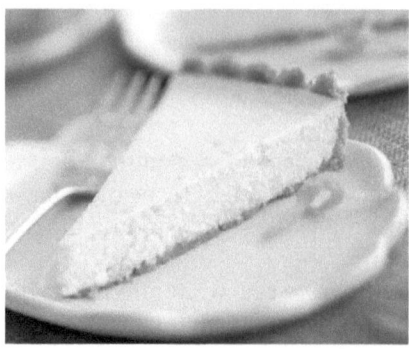

Ingredients

For the Crust

- 1 cup pitted dates (soaked and drained)
- 1 cup shredded coconut
- 1 cup cashews
- 1 tsp vanilla extract

For the Filling

- 3 extra-large oranges
- 1 cup fat-free plain Greek yogurt
- 2 tsp vanilla extract
- 12 tsp stevia

Method

1. In a bowl, mix the dates, coconut, cashews, and vanilla crust ingredients together. Press the crust mixture into a greased muffin tin. Place the filling ingredients into a food process until a smooth consistency is achieved. Pour the filling evenly onto each of the crusts, and freeze overnight.

115. Coconut Cream Pie Bars

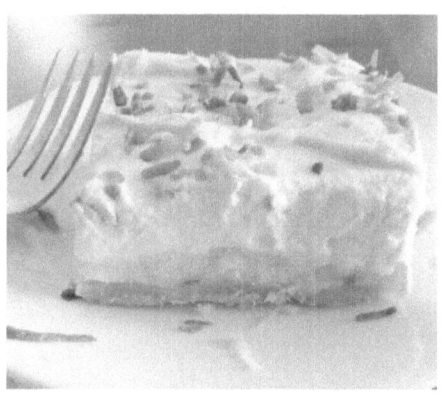

Ingredients

For the Crust

- ½ cup shredded coconut
- 1 cup chopped cashews
- 1 cup pitted dates (soaked and drained)
- 2 tbsp. water

For the Filling

- ½ cup almond butter
- ¼ cup low-fat coconut milk
- 1 tbsp. vanilla
- ⅓ cup shredded coconut
- 6 tsp stevia

Method

1. In a bowl, combine filling ingredients almond butter, coconut milk, vanilla, coconut, and stevia. Mix well and set aside. In a separate bowl, combine the crust ingredients coconut, cashews, dates, and water in a bowl and mix well. In a greased 8x8 tin press the crust into the tin evenly.

2. Grease an 8×8 baking pan or glass dish with a healthy oil. Spoon filling evenly into the tin, sprinkle coconut on top, and freeze overnight.

116. Berry Pudding

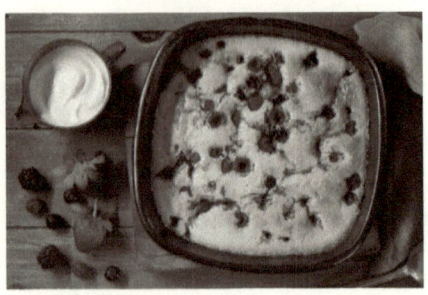

Ingredients

- 1 (1 lbs.) loaf Brioche or Challah Bread (cut into 1" slices)
- 2 pints Strawberries (quartered)
- 2 pints Blueberries
- 2 pints Blackberries
- 2 pints Raspberries
- 1 cup Sugar
- 1 Vanilla Bean (split lengthwise)
- 6 Tbsps. Butter
- ½ tsp Cinnamon

Method

1. Line a pan with plastic wrap. Place pan on a baking sheet. In a pot, mix together all berries, ½ cup water, and 1 cup sugar. Simmer 10 minutes, stirring often. Set aside.

2. Spread butter onto bread slices. Mix 2 tablespoons sugar with cinnamon. Sprinkle over buttered bread. Drizzle ½ cup berry sauce in bottom of lined pan.

3. Arrange a single layer of bread slices in pan. Pour 1 ½ cups berry sauce over bread. Repeat this layering until ingredients are used up. Cover with plastic. Set a plate in the pan and weigh it down with heavy cans. Chill 1 hour.

Health Benefits of Berries

Improves brain health and cognitive function. Help control appetite and manage weight. Helps prevent age-related illnesses like Alzheimer's.

117. Fruit Cobbler

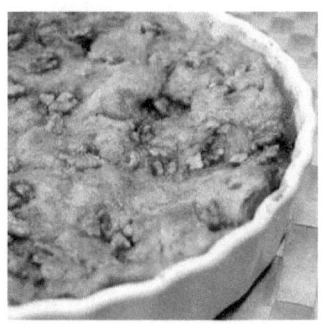

Ingredients

- 4 cups Nectarines (peeled, sliced)
- 1-pint Raspberries
- 2/3 cup Sugar
- 1 ¼ cup Flour
- ½ cup Cornmeal
- 6 Tbsps. Buttermilk
- 5 Tbsps. Butter (sliced)
- 2 Tbsps. Cornstarch
- 1 Tbsp. Raw Sugar
- 1 Tbsp. Fresh Lemon Juice
- 2 tsp Baking Powder
- ¾ tsp Salt
- ½ tsp Baking Soda

Method

1. Preheat oven to 375°F. In a bowl, toss together raspberries, nectarines, cornstarch, juice, ¼ teaspoon salt, and 1/3 cup sugar. Add mixture to a greased baking dish.

2. In another bowl, whisk together remaining sugar, cornmeal, baking powder, baking soda, flour, and ½ teaspoon salt. Add flour mixture to food processor with butter. Pulse until dough forms pea-sized pieces.

3. Add buttermilk. Pulse until combined. Measure out 1/3 cup portions of dough to create 10 round biscuits. Place biscuits on top of fruit mixture in baking dish. Lightly press biscuits down with fingers. Sprinkle the top with raw sugar. Bake 50 minutes.

Health Benefits of Nectarines

High in antioxidants. Helps maintain collagen and prevent wrinkles. Improves digestion and helps weight loss.

Final Words

I would like to thank you for downloading my book and I hope I have been able to help you and educate you about something new.

If you have enjoyed this book and would like to share your positive thoughts, could you please take 30 seconds of your time to go back and give me a review on my Amazon book page!

I greatly appreciate seeing these reviews because it helps me share my hard work!

Again, thank you and I wish you all the best with your cooking journey!

Last Chance to Get YOUR Bonus!

FOR A LIMITED TIME ONLY – Get Olivia's best-selling book *"The #1 Cookbook: Over 170+ of the Most Popular Recipes Across 7 Different Cuisines!"* absolutely FREE!

Readers have absolutely loved this book because of the wide variety of recipes. It is highly recommended you check these recipes out and see what you can add to your home menu!

Once again, as a big thank-you for downloading this book, I'd like to offer it to you *100% FREE for a LIMITED TIME ONLY!*

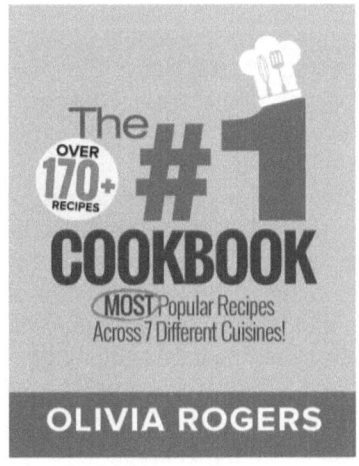

Get your free copy at:

TheMenuAtHome.com/Bonus

Disclaimer

This book and related site provides recipe and food advice in an informative and educational manner only, with information that is general in nature and that is not specific to you, the reader. The contents of this book and related site are intended to assist you and other readers in your personal efforts. Consult your physician or nutritionist regarding the applicability of any information provided in our information to you.

Nothing in this book should be construed as personal advice or diagnosis, and must not be used in this manner. The information provided about conditions is general in nature. This information does not cover all possible uses, actions, precautions, side-effects, or interactions of medicines, or medical procedures. The information in this site should not be considered as complete and does not cover all diseases, ailments, physical conditions, or their treatment.

No Warranties: The authors and publishers don't guarantee or warrant the quality, accuracy, completeness, timeliness, appropriateness or suitability of the information in this book, or of any product or services referenced by this site.

The information in this site is provided on an "as is" basis and the authors and publishers make no representations or warranties of any kind with respect to this information. This site may contain inaccuracies, typographical errors, or other errors.

Liability Disclaimer: The publishers, authors, and other parties involved in the creation, production, provision of information, or delivery of this site specifically disclaim any responsibility, and shall not be held liable for any damages, claims, injuries, losses, liabilities, costs, or obligations including any direct, indirect, special, incidental, or consequences damages (collectively known as "Damages") whatsoever and howsoever caused, arising out of, or in connection with the use or misuse of the site and the information contained within it, whether such Damages arise in contract, tort, negligence, equity, statute law, or by way of other legal theory.

www.ingramcontent.com/pod-product-compliance
Lightning Source LLC
Chambersburg PA
CBHW031124080526
44587CB00011B/1104